The Mighty Cobra and The Pink Rabbit

To order additional copies, please contact us.
BookSurge, LLC
www.booksurge.com
1-866-308-6235
orders@booksurge.com

MISS PINK

THE MIGHTY COBRA AND THE PINK RABBIT

2006

The Mighty Cobra and The Pink Rabbit

I Dedicate This Book To:

Yogiraj Bikram Choudhury

***

Mrs. RAC Webster

***

Barbara Bohrer

***

My Prince

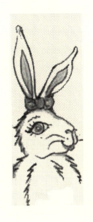

PROLOGUE

Once upon a time, there was a girl raised in a happy house filled with joy.
(Though her hair was cut too short and she was often mistaken for a boy.)

Like her clan, she was kind hearted and dressed with flair.
Like all the girls in her family, her body was shaped like a pear.

She never once thought that being a pear was necessarily bad,
Until authority figures said things that made her oh-so-sad.

Her ballet teacher told her she'd never be able to take a pointe class.
"The tutus, my dear, are not wide enough to cover your ass."

The drill team instructor said she'd sure win the top spirit prize.
"However, we can't cheer to victory with those big thighs."

The broadcasting dean said her writing style was profound, uncanny.
"However the television screen is simply too small for your fanny."

She went through life, day after day, feeling quite odd.
"I've only got this one," she'd think, "this one pear-shaped bod."

Her romantic life often went from mediocre to bad to worse.
To heal, she'd cozy up with Bailey's and pen mean-spirited verse.

The tall trust fund frat boy stole her heart and then turned snide.
"I adore your brains and smile but loathe your backside."

The banker sent flowers and notes, not aware he would offend
When he whispered, "I have a fetish for you and your giant rear end."

The one with broad shoulders had a rod that just wouldn't get hard.
"I'm sorry my sweets, but every time I see your thighs, I think of lard."

She kept going on, sometimes quite woefully, down life's path.
Taking comfort in knowing she wasn't as sad as Sylvia Plath.

It made her angry; this pear shape wasn't exactly her choice.
Over time, she garnered great attention for having a great voice.

Hiding behind the smokescreen of the radio dial,
She finally found her passion, her reason to smile.

At home, though, she would run and swim,
Hoping one day to simply morph into thin.

A dear friend Helen cajoled and begged, "You've got to give yoga a try."
"I can't, I can't, I'm such a stiff little pear, stretching makes me cry."

She started with yoga made gentle for those over 65.
It hurt, she was sore, she limped—this was no way to thrive.

She tried again, at a place where they hopped and spun.
However, the 6 A.M. wakeup calls were simply no fun.

About to give up, she went to a studio that promised she'd sweat a lot.
For the first time in her life, the shape of her body she simply forgot.

The heat made her sweat and detox and become loose.
One day she said to herself: "My, I've got a nice little caboose."

She transformed, she dripped, to new heights she did reach.
Knowing by the tenth class, this yoga she had to teach.

In order to teach, you get a blessing, an official stamp
By surviving Bikram's infamous nine-week yoga boot camp.

She was hooked, her skin glowed, she had become a regular yoga junky.
Though she did fret about the voice in her head, a mean-spirited monkey.

As our pear grew up surrounded by a family well-rounded,
Bikram's physical feats, by age four, simply astounded.

As our pear was told, "Your body won't do, that's impossible, never, never;"
Bikram was told, "Your body is your ticket, you'll be great forever and ever."

So our two opposites came together one year, a little like The Odd Couple,
She being doubtful and stiff, he dynamic and supple.

They butted heads, they disagreed, there were insults, and someone came undone. Who?
To find out, you'll have to start at the beginning, on page one.

MONDAY 3 JANUARY 2005

We had a great Christmas. Just got back last night from the east coast wedding—hard to imagine that baby Amanda is married now. She looked really great; actually everyone did. My two aunts returned to Weight Watchers after a 10-month hiatus and dragged the bride-to-be with them. It is what we do, my family—we weigh. And we struggle with weight. We talk carbs and goal weights and we occasionally walk away from Weight Watchers to give Jenny Craig a try. If Jenny lets us down, we'll toy with the Sonoma diet and reminisce about the Scarsdale diet. Sometimes we'll muse to each other, sure wish we could lose those last damn ten pounds. Sitting around the dining room table, someone eventually sighs and says, "We have just got to watch every bite. If we don't, we'll end up looking like Aunt Katherine."

Poor, sweet, maligned Aunt Katherine. No one knew for sure what she did weigh. She was quite large and rumor had it that she needed truck scales to get an accurate number. She was at least 400 pounds, maybe 430. Jolly, funny woman with diabetes, and a penchant for whiskey and dark chocolate. I always liked Aunt Katherine; she was funny and a bit gassy and swore like a sailor.

This is a momentous family gathering for me. The last time I went to a family thing—my uncle's funeral, I think—I was trapped in a torturous two-year divorce process, I still hadn't recovered from losing my dot-com job, and my dog was still incontinent. The interactions with my family were pretty brief.

"Still living with him, huh?"

"Yup."

"Still haven't gotten that divorce yet, huh?"

"Nope."

"Still living in that old farmhouse?"

"Yup."

"Didja try that bean casserole? Good, huh?"

"Yup."

That was then.

Now I'm back and I've got buckets of news. The biggest news item is The New Husband. Bad enough that I'm the first kid in the family to divorce, but then, to the shock of my nice Midwestern family, not only did I remarry—I met The New Husband at a bar! And not just at a bar, but at a singles party! And then, I eloped with him, practically the next week! (We did wait twelve months, but my family tends toward long engagements.)

Not only do I have The New Husband in tow, but we've had a pretty eventful year: he moved in with me while we finished up the renovations at his house—and—I got accepted into yoga college.

I will admit I was sort of nervous telling my family about the yoga thing. They are quite hardy, the family. They have manly jobs involving trucks and construction and farming thingamabobs. They are the sort of men who like pie at lunch—and the women who make those pies from scratch. The men hunt; the women quilt.

My branch of the family tree is a bit of an anomaly. For starters, my parents actually left the little town and moved to a big town. My dad has had suit-and-briefcase jobs and my mom has not had to make a lunch pail for him. My dad often jokes that if he had to actually go out and kill his dinner, he'd happily be a vegetarian.

I took my parents' small-town escape a step further and I moved to the giant swarm of New York City. I dabbled in public relations and Wall Street.

In short, our hardy hunting trunk of the family tree already thinks my branch is a bit alien. The very fact that we have not driven a tractor in our sheltered lives makes us veritable circus freaks. Adding yoga to the mix? Heaven only knows.

I can't entirely blame it on them, though, you know, this perceived yoga-aversion.

The thing is, I'm no bendy twig girl. I'm a pear-shaped, middle-aged woman with wobbly thighs and an ongoing concern that the new jeans/bathing suit/lighting/hairstyle/purse/lip gloss (fill in the blank) makes my butt look fat.

As I wandered through the divorce maze, I was battling some sadness. The doctors were quick to throw an antidepressant prescription at me, but I felt that I had earned my crying jags. I wanted to be certain that I wallowed in my unhappiness. I'm not sure why, but I think mostly I feared that chemically induced happiness might backfire and I'd just end up with chemically induced stupidity or, worse yet, an odd Stepford-Wife-ish appreciation of my smelly, flatulent ex-husband.

My therapist gave me a list of "things to do when you are depressed." The list went like this: establish network of friends for support, increase physical activity, eat healthier foods, find enjoyable hobbies, see a mental health professional, meditate, do yoga.

Being an overachiever, I found a way to get most of that list covered in one fell swoop. I joined a synchronized swim team, thereby increasing my activity, making new friends, establishing a hobby and eating healthier. I bought meditation tapes and listened to them with a closed and suspicious mind.

Yoga?

No way.

Therapist and I had an agreement: if I did everything on the list for six months, she wouldn't push the pills.

And the therapist stood her ground—everything on the list, including the bleeping yoga. Again, the joy of multitasking struck. One of my synchronized swim teammates taught yoga. And not yoga, but easy-peasy (to my mind) yoga: gentle yoga for seniors. I cringe to admit this, but here ya go: I thought maybe I could out bend at least the elderly. (That's awful, isn't it? But I was quite desperate.)

All I got from the senior yoga class was free coffee and an intensified pent-up loathing of flexible people. Even 70-year-old widows recovering from double hip replacement were better at yoga than I was.

Oddly, handsome Prince was one factor in my abrupt change of heart. An ex-girlfriend of his convinced him to try Bikram's hot yoga and Prince thought I'd like it. Initially, being a slightly competitive snot, I thought, oh no, I will not take up her hobby. But Prince is an earthy sort and his enthusiasm for Bikram's yoga struck a chord.

I'm looking over our family's sea of familiar faces and am so happy to see Prince working the crowd. He's normally a pretty quiet person, but he seems to flit with ease through my gaggles of gawking relatives. Prince has quite an advantage: he has gone hunting. The relatives collectively cheered on hearing this—he's not a subway-riding city freak, he's not a prep school rube who can't tell a duck from a goose—no no! He's a regular animal-stalking guy.

I slip away and find Aunt Mary Jane. She was the stricter aunt when I was growing up; she's got a wicked stern eyebrow arch that'll scare any child into not only stopping what they are doing, but also erasing the desire to ever be naughty again. I figure if I get the yoga news past her, I'm into smooth water.

I tell her my yoga college news and her eyes get real big and she says, "Didja really?"

She clucks her tongue and shakes her head side to side and whispers, "Is that something The New Husband made ya do?".

I told her about my gentle yoga attempts and how, the last time she saw me, I disliked yoga as much as I dislike flossing.

But then last year happened. She nodded her chin and up and down strongly.

If we were a Southern Baptist family, she'd follow the chin nodding with "Tell it to the man, sister." Instead, we are Northern Lutherans, and chin nodding is as vigorous as it gets for our clan.

I don't have to explain "last year happened" to her. She knows. She sat by the phone like everyone else in the family.

***

So I'm newly-divorced and I go to a singles party and I meet Prince. We are just five weeks into a new fairy tale-ish romance, I'm freelance writing and Prince poaches eggs for me on the weekends and then, blam. I'm doubled over in pain, Prince is driving at warp speed to get me to the emergency room. Pain like I've never ever felt, white cold pain, the kind that takes the strength out of your legs, the kind that makes you mewl like a kitten, vicious angry pain that gives morphine a run for its money.

Sonogram shows an ovarian cyst has ruptured. No real known cause or cure, really. Just ride it out.

(And let me tell you, there's nothing like your new man holding your hand through an emergency vaginal sonogram to fling a dewy relationship to an entirely new level.)

The Monday after the ER visit, I go to my gynecologist for a follow up. She does a full exam and checks the breasts while we are at it. Her eyes darken and I'm given an emergency mammogram slip and the following Tuesday, the mammogram reveals two cysts on the left breast.

The mammogram center is really nice and posh and they do a sonogram just to be sure and they humor me when I say I want both breasts sonogrammed for the sake of symmetry. Sonogram reveals calcifications in the right breast. Calcifications are little sandy bits that usually hang out together and then often turn into a cancer of some form. My mum is a feisty breast cancer survivor, so part of me feels resigned to it all and part of me is glad I know the terminology.

Not only do I know the lingo, I also know that when the doctor's office says you need to come in the following day, it isn't to unkink an insurance issue. I assume the worst, immediately go to Google and research wig options. If I'm going to go bald from chemo, I'd rather harvest my own hair than glue someone else's on my head.

The doctor has good news. The right breast calcifications were all sucked up through the mini- Hoover vacuum for the biopsy. They are fine; benign; noncancerous. Phew.

The reason the doctor wants to see me is that my pap smear came back showing abnormal growth, probably not a good kind of growth. There's some kind of lab holiday and then some kind of snarl with the new patient privacy laws, so I have to wait 11 agonizing days to hear the newest biopsy news.

Eleven days. Two hundred and sixty-one hours, at least half of which were spent staring at a stale pack of Marlboro Light 100s, desperately wishing I hadn't quit smoking. I drank a lot of Bailey's Irish Cream in those 11 days. On the morning of the twelfth day, the doctor informed me that there was a cervical polyp, a little bump, and again, the biopsy Hoover vac sucked it right out. Benign. Okay. Time to throw out the wig brochures.

I vowed that cold November morning—I did—I swore to myself that I would be so nice to my body from that point forward. Well, right after Thanksgiving. Well, okay, right after Christmas. The holidays would be about rejoicing and celebrating and then in January—as long as it wasn't bad weather—then I would live every single day to the fullest, I would worship my body in new ways, I'd eat organic leafy greens and moisturize more often and be better about taking a multivitamin.

I blink, and it is April. Bada-bing, my six-month follow up appointments are looming on the calendar. All the gals—both breasts, the cervix, the ovaries—need to be prodded again, to make sure no weeds have sprouted. I know I cannot sit through another agonizing week, I will surely pull my hair out strand by strand, staring at the phone, waiting.

I'm not sure what I will do, but I know that I have gained a few pounds in the past six months. There I am, bouncing on my ergonomic ball, Googling to see if there's such a thing as low-cal Bailey's. Bing. I get an e-mail from someone I haven't heard from in a goodly 10 years. College pal Nicole drops me a note and writes quite glowingly about Bikram Yoga.

Maybe Prince's ex-girlfriend was on to something good. Nicole is a perfectly sweet and wonderful sorority little sister – she wouldn't lead me astray.

***

"Say that name again; how did you pronounce it?" Aunt Mary Jane asks.

"Beak, likes a bird's beak and then rum, like, you know, rum."

"Is that a person or a place?"

"It is a person."

"Is he one of those Buddha statues?"

"No, actually Bikram is alive and well."

I tell Aunt Mary Jane that I hadn't really heard of him either until my friend emailed.

Well, prior to Prince and prior to Nicole, I vaguely remember reading a newspaper article a while back about some kind of copyright issue. But that was about the extent of my knowledge.

Aunt Shirley—Mary Jane's older sister—walks over in her crisp and decided way.

"What are you two talking about over here?"

I tell her Bikram, and explain that it is hot yoga.

"How hot does it get?"

She whistles as she pulls in air through her lips. "One hundred and five degrees? Is that safe? When we brought in the baby chicks for the feed store, I think we kept it right around 95 degrees. Too hot was dangerous for the chicks. You think this is really safe?"

A small crowd had formed. My family, we are lemmings. We follow each other and when more than two lemmings are together, the others panic, feel left out, and flock.

One uncle wanted to know if I wore baggy pants like Gandhi. A sweet cousin in her 20s said her church told her she wouldn't be allowed to organize a yoga class as the minister believed that yoga belonged to Hindus, not Lutherans.

There are now a good dozen or so family members gathered 'round, full of questions. That's one thing I adore about my family—our unending curiosity.

Finally one of my cousins blurts out, "I thought ya had to be skinny to do that weird yoga stuff." Half question, half accusation.

Another jocular wedding guest (and, let's be frank, jocularity was brought on by seven Pabst beers) says that yoga isn't so much about weight as it is about wrapping your legs around your neck. That comment ignites a hearty round of people wanting a demonstration. I half-imagine them waving giant foam hands in the air, it has become as boisterous as a Super Bowl playoff game.

I decline their offer for proof of my yoganess. I say graciously that I am not warmed up. I have barely finished the sentence, and there's unprecedented laughing, and not jolly laughter now, no, no, we have slid past bemused and right into the slippery sarcasm slope.

My round German/French/Swiss/American Indian mutt family is snorting and clapping and laughing as though it was the funniest thing they'd heard all month, if not all decade.

One barrel-chested uncle, red faced from laughter, said, "She isn't warmed up yet."

Barrel uncle pauses dramatically, to make sure we all notice that he's put giant neon finger quotes around the words "warmed up" as though I were fumbling for an excuse. I really do not like finger quotes.

He continues, he's on a roll, barrel uncle is. "Didn't ya say it is hot yoga? They will eat you alive at this hot yoga college."

The slight advantage to all the yoga joshing is that my family has, albeit briefly, lost their focus on my sweet new husband, Prince. Prince is busy trying to hide his shock at our family shenanigans. Prince is, after all, a civilian. That's the family's code word for those lucky people who are rumored to just eat what they want and don't gain weight or need to try to lose weight. Civilians wear the same size clothing year round and do not attend meetings involving public weigh-ins. Civilians, in near-mythic status in our round little family, have a good and blessed and easy life.

Thinking about the family from Prince's point of view makes me see, probably for the first time, that the chatter in my head about my body, my thighs, my arse, my scales, my exercise—all this chatter is not entirely my doing.

I used to worry that all the thoughts in my head were signs of mental illness. I was relieved to learn that Buddhists refer to fleeting, zipping, tripping thoughts as monkey mind. It makes sense! Those random musings do feel like mischievous monkeys. Over the years, my mind monkeys have taken on distinct personalities.

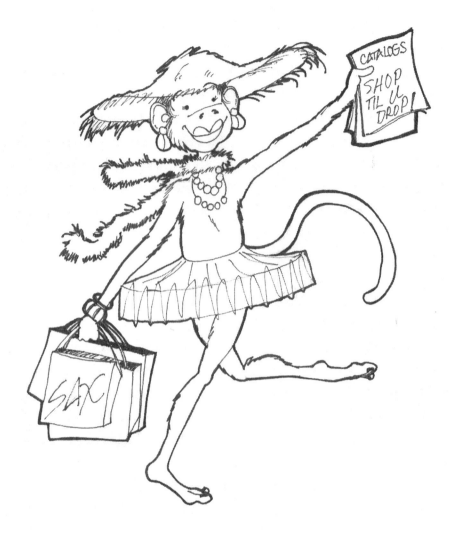

There's Shopping Monkey. She likes wearing a pink tutu and a large-brimmed feather-adorned hat and big gaudy necklaces. She's always wearing way too much lipstick; no doubt leftovers from all her stops at the makeup counter. One hand is loaded with shopping bags, the other has a fistful of catalogs.

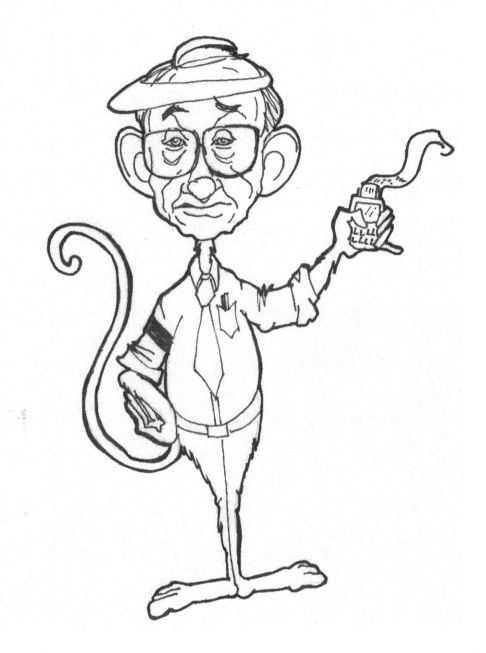

On most days, Shopping Monkey is locked in mortal combat with Money Monkey. Money Monkey looks a little like Alan Greenspan and when the two of them start chasing each other in circles—she wants the new suede moccasins with pink trim, he's insisting the money is better left in an interest-bearing savings account—well, who really can concentrate on anything with all that going on?

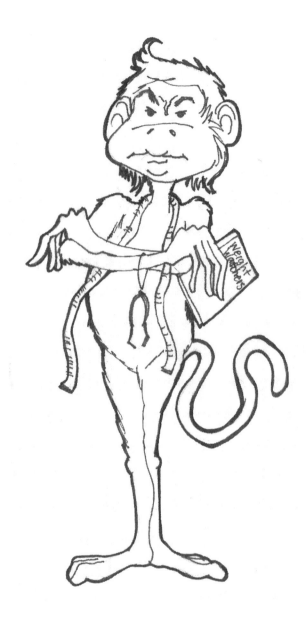

Pudge Monkey has the pinched face of an angry, unforgiving, constipated nun. She's got a measuring tape around her neck. She always has a body fat tester on hand, which reminds me of a nutcracker, which usually makes me hungry if I think about it long enough. She also religiously clutches a well-worn copy of the Weight Watchers food guide and a picture of me, taken when I weighed 117 pounds and the only picture that I like of myself.

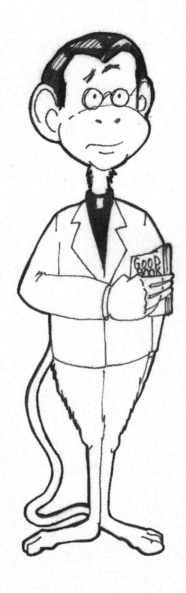

Morality Monkey is mostly silent. He looks like a good Irish Catholic priest, little round glasses, well-kept grooming. He almost always has a book in his right hand. He's got a velvet-smooth voice. And while he isn't as busy as the other monkeys, when he does speak, he hones in on the issue at hand succinctly and with kindness.

When I wake up in the morning, the first thing I do is look in the mirror to see if I still look, well, you know, not-so-thin. I think a lot of mornings, I'm secretly hoping that I'll look in the mirror and say "Oh my gosh, I'm not fat anymore!" Pudge Monkey is there every morning to keep me humble, remind me of my sins. Pudge Monkey, however, gets quiet when the scales show more than a one-pound drop. That's when Shopping Monkey takes over.

So I realized, in the middle of Amanda's wedding reception, that I didn't just wake up one day and have fully dressed monkeys running around in my head. No no no. Nature, nurture. Some of this was homegrown, nurtured like a small houseplant, seeds of doubt buried in layers of family routine, watered with folklore, basking in the warmth of a cup of low-calorie nonfat hot chocolate and a three-ounce serving of unbuttered popcorn.

It's slightly embarrassing to be afraid of an imaginary nun-looking monkey—but she's my biggest worry about going to yoga boot camp. I'm going to spend 10, 12 hours a day in a mirrored room surrounded, no doubt, by lithe young limber bodies. I feel pretty sure I'll be okay doing the yoga. But is my mind healthy enough? I'm not entirely sure.

WEDNESDAY 5 JANUARY

Have to make time today for my annual rune reading. Small velvet bag containing the rune tiles and then a sweet little blue book—author Ralph Blum. That one super-psychotic college friend of mine gave it to me as a gift 20 years ago. Every year, I think I should get a new set, maybe it has her mental illness stowed in it. But a ritual is a ritual. That, and there's a rumor that if you buy yourself your own runes, you will have bad luck. Who needs that?

Anyway, the runes seem much more legit than tarot cards. Or maybe they are just easier to read. They are small white stone tiles, about the size of a Mahjong square. And unless I am drunk when I do the reading, they are always correct. I always do the six-tile layout—it's nice and comprehensive. Goes to the immediate past, into now, immediate future, foundation of the issue at hand, obstacle, and outcome. For this year—couldn't be more perfect for a gal on the eve of a new adventure.

The Immediate Past--Opening Rune. I've got to gladly give up the old life, live empty for a while, wait for a new way to become illuminated. (Put duct tape over Pudge Monkey's blabbing mouth. Time to think like a Civilian.)

The Now--Journey Rune. What looks like failure is actually a rerouting possibility. (I just lost the most recent freelancing gig, which hurts financially, but allows me to focus on yoga, yoga, yoga.)

The Immediate Future--Self Rune. If I want to know what enemy to slay, look inside. My internal enemy is a reflection of that which I have long recognized in myself. (Take that Pudge Monkey!)

The Foundation--Fertility Rune. I can now complete. The completion will bring me a new beginning. I'm no longer gestating—time to enter the delivery room. (Not sure, but sounds exciting.)

The Potential Obstacle--Growth Rune. Aspects of my internal character will interfere with the growth of my new life, if I let them. (Reason #74 to knock out Pudge Monkey.)

Best Possible Outcome--Warrior Rune. Stay out of my own way and let the will of heavens flow through me. Look within to best deal with the very deepest needs of my nature. (What are my deepest needs, really? Shopping Monkey believes those cellulite-melting pants are my primary deepest need and I think she's right.)

FRIDAY 7 JANUARY

I've reread my runes and I'm afraid I'm overlooking one giant problem. Me and authority figures.

I also realized I don't know very much at all about this man that I've now pledged my troth to, career-wise. Maybe this is how women feel when they first find out they are pregnant. There's a glow and a blush and then a sinking sense of, "Oh, crud, what have I gotten myself into?"

Spent a lot of time on Google these past couple of days, trying to get a better sense of this Bikram man. His thumbnail biography reads like a fable. Born in Calcutta. Started yoga at age four, under the tutelage of a famous man, Bishnu Ghosh. World Yoga Champion three years running. Weight lifting accident at age 17 destroyed his knee. Doctors told him he'd never walk again.

Bikram returned to his mentor, Bishnu, for guidance. Some say he insisted on being carried back to Bishnu. The two of them yoga-ed like mad for six months and then—voila!— he can walk again.

Not only can he walk, he goes straight to the Olympics. Literally. He competed in the 1964 Olympics in Tokyo.

And then he's teaching yoga to Jane Fonda and Shirley MacLaine in Beverly Hills. USA Today ran an article on Bikram in early 2000—accompanied with a picture of him standing on a student in a backbend.

Bikram told ABC News that he's "bulletproof, waterproof, fireproof, windproof, money-proof, sex-proof."

Yoga Journal wrote an article headlined "Yoga's Bad Boy" with the subtitle reading "He sells Rolls Royces in Beverly Hills, hobnobs with Hollywood glitterati, and claims that he alone teaches true Hatha Yoga."

That takes a lot of nerve, telling the Yoga Journal that he's the only one doing it right. Not only that, he told the reporter that nonBikram yoga teachers are "like circus clowns . . . [they don't] know what the hell they are doing."

The Economist called him "The Litigious Yogi."

And Business 2.0 titled their Bikram profile "Yogis Behaving Badly." He told that reporter that he's like Jesus Christ and that he can cure every disease known. When the reporter dared to question how he could make such claims, Bikram replied, "Because I have balls like atom bombs, two of them, 100 megatons each. Nobody fucks with me."

That last sentence strikes a chord.

Reminds me of my band director in high school. The band director who once threw his baton and his sheet music and then the entire podium at me during practice. Claimed I was sharp. I knew I wasn't sharp—just that as the piccolo, you tend to be the highest note in the band and the easiest to blame. Plus which, I was directly in front of him and the easiest to throw things at.

The podium-tossing incident happened about two weeks before a big and important concert. So I went on strike; I refused to play until he apologized. I remember talking with my guidance counselor about the podium tossing and the counselor asking if I had had "authority figure issues." I thought back to the kindergarten lunch lady and the third grade recess monitor and the seventh grade social studies guy and I lied and said "No."

The counselor advised that I apologize to the band director, which seemed obscene—he could have injured me! He could have poked my eye out! Why should I apologize to him?

For two very long weeks, I sat in band every day, fingering all the notes to my solos, just refusing to blow air into my piccolo and produce sound.

The day of the performance, the band director pulled me into his office, closed the door, pulled down the green shade over the door window and said, "What is it going to take to get you to play?"

"An apology."

"Okay, you can apologize any time you want."

"No, sorry, sir. I need for you to apologize to me. I had a bruise on my knee for nearly a week from the podium. And I wasn't sharp. The oboe was flat."

"I will not apologize to you. You play the piccolo, for god's sake!"

"So if I played tuba you'd apologize?"

"Yes. No. That's not what I meant. I am the teacher. I have won awards. No one ever, ever—and I mean ever—fucks with me."

It was the first time I had heard that eff word and I was anxious to get to the dictionary.

With that giant proclamation of his, I turned around and walked out of the room. He followed me, slightly panicked, grabbed my arm and asked what would happen during all those solos he had given me? Would there just be silence? Would I honestly ruin a performance just on pride?

In my heart of hearts, I thought, nah, I love performing. I'll just put a scare into him.

That night, the band director and I were behind the curtains, waiting for our cue. Since I was first chair flute (and famed piccolo soloist!), the tradition called for both of us to walk onto the stage together. It was a point of no return for both of us.

"So, little miss piccolo—what do I have to do to get you to play?"

"Say you are sorry."

"For what! I'm your band director. I am never fucked with, kid, never!"

"Okay."

"Okay what?"

"Okay, I believe you. I understand."

"God, you are impossible. Fine."

The emcee is announcing the band, the crowd is applauding, the curtains are opening. I saw a bead of sweat run from his left temple, heading straight for his ear.

"Sorry."

"Excuse me, sir?"

"How many times do I have to say it? Sorry damnit."

"You have to mean it. And you have to use it in a sentence. And right now, you don't mean it. You are just saying it to get me on stage."

"You are a fucking piece of work, kid."

There's a long silence and we are staring at each other and I think about the phrase "authority issue" and I think that, yes, this is an issue, but I've got to start defending my own honor and now's a perfect time.

He clears his throat and shifts his weight back and forth, left foot, right foot, left foot, right foot.

"Listen. I am sorry. Really. I truly am sorry."

"That wasn't so hard, was it? Thank you. Apology accepted."

I think my game plan will simply be to avoid this Bikram guy. One thing to be a sassy 16-year-old gal with a band director over a barrel. Quite another ball game to be a grown adult, embarking on a new career, investing my life savings into this education. I will simply fade into the background, I will be like those fish that change color, I will vanish before his eyes.

That way, he can use the power of his mighty two-ton balls on some other poor schmuck with authority issues.

SATURDAY 15 JANUARY

# of consecutive days doing yoga: 13
# of days until yoga boot camp: 85

At the beginning of each year, my yoga studio, the Sweatbox, hosts a 30-day yoga challenge. Do yoga for 30 days in a row. There are two owners of the Sweatbox—Laura and Frankie. They both agreed that doing the challenge would be a great way for me to get ready for the yoga teacher training that starts in April (now less than three months away).

Teacher training will be 99 classes in 9 weeks, which seems unfathomably daunting. But everyone has got to start somewhere. Right?

Plus which, I read on one yoga studio's website that doing a 30-day yoga challenge will "forever change your body, forever change your life."

I asked Frankie last week if that was true, the forever-change thing. She cocked her chin 30 degrees to the left, the same way my poodle Becky does when she's taking something under advisement. She laughed and said, "Well, I don't know what you are expecting, but it isn't like your hair will change color, that kind of change."

I felt slightly deflated. I had hoped Frankie would say, "Oh, yes. Every single person that has done a 30-day yoga challenge walks away with dimple-free thighs and the winning Lotto ticket."

Frankie will be my boss when I come home from training, so I'm a little more careful these days in what I blurt out in front of her. I didn't dare admit that I hope to slay the monkeys shrieking in my head. And I also don't want to admit that I desperately want a mid-body transplant. Really. Just from knees to belly button, if that region could be less lumpy and bumpy, that is about 80 percent of what I really desire from all this yoga stuff.

So I thought, okay, Mr. Bikram. You got it. Consider yourself challenged. This body won't change one iota. I've done everything I can think of in terms of exercise. Synchronized swimming, weight lifting, hell, spent two years training for the New York City Marathon—and through it all, my thighs stayed stubbornly wibbly and dimply.

Bikram promises in his book that the Awkward Pose—which involves sitting down on an imaginary chair—he promises this will take care of cellulite. So far, I'm not feeling that love.

Since I've decided to be an uber overachiever, I've committed to not just a 30-day or 60-day challenge. No way! I'm going for broke, 90 days in a row. I figure it'll be a multitasking experience—I can melt my thighs away, lose the 10 to 12 pounds that I lied about on my teacher training application, and shift my shape a bit.

Now that I've declared, "I want to teach yoga," I've really started to fret about my round little body. I don't think it is the right type, you know, to stand in front of students and teach.

But on the way back home from Christmas, the bag screeners at Newark Airport were complaining about how much their necks and shoulders ached. Before Prince had put his shoes back on, I had three security guys doing a really nice Eagle Pose. And they were so happy, they had such changed faces after two sets of Eagle. Just two minutes earlier, they were crabby, frowny-faced, overworked, under-appreciated employees. Two sets of Eagle, they are hugging me and waving good-bye and swinging their arms in circles in amazement at how a simple, quick posture could bring them so much relief.

I muttered to myself, "Well, then. This is what you were meant to do." I simply couldn't fathom a life of not teaching yoga.

Ever since I got my yoga college acceptance news in November, the Monkeys have been in full swing. Shopping Monkey is obsessed with finding the perfect yoga shorts that will hide my lumpy thighs. Money Monkey's adding machine is running day and night. Pudge Monkey is in full Code Red, shrieking and throwing rotten banana chunks to get my attention. Over and over, Pudge reminds me that I have gained weight, that my summer Capris aren't even zipping any more, that the news executive said I was too fat for television and the cheerleading coach said I was too fat to be cheery and that fabulously wealthy guy broke up with me because my thighs were too ucky for his tastes. So it goes, she's got a long list, Pudge Monkey, of all the times my weight has blocked me from what was supposed to be mine.

Morality Monkey is growing concerned about the slight, shall we say, discrepancies on my yoga boot camp application.

Not really fibs though, more like slight mistruths.

I went to the Bikram Yoga website to fill out the application in November. The website's instructions were to fill out the form online, click submit, and then print it out and mail it to them. So for starters, I did honestly think this was a work-in-progress kind of thing. Fill it out, dabble around with the essay, print it out and then make changes and find an envelope big enough.

So my first slight mistruth was this checkbox that said I promised I was ready, willing, and able to study at least two hours per day in addition to the daily schedule. I chuckled to myself, knowing full well that there was no way I'd go through a bruising yoga boot camp day and then come home and study too.

Yoga teacher training begins each day at 9:30 A.M. with a 90-minute Bikram Yoga class. One hour for lunch. Then five hours of lectures, anatomy classes, studying each posture. Straight from that into the 5:00 P.M. yoga class. A little over an hour for dinner. And then— from 8:00 P.M. until midnight—lectures! I'm supposed to study until 2:00 or 3:00 in the morning? I think not.

One giant relief is that the morning class isn't at the crack of dawn. Seems like lots of yoga zealots are into that, the sunrise thing. Not this chick.

I will admit—all my family's initial reactions to yoga weren't that different from mine. I had always thought yoga types were granola-crunching tie-dye fanatics who shunned deodorant for political reasons.

Shopping Monkey rallied and quickly helped me see that yoga could be what I made it to be. Shopping Monkey quickly located really precious (and, in some cases, really spendy) yoga clothing online. I'm quite convinced that my $79 pants make me look at least 12 pounds thinner than my $7 pants.

I'm not sure how I will keep ahead of all the book studying, but I am pretty sure I will have matching outfits for each part of the day. I do believe that 90 percent of all social blending issues stem from proper attire.

The second slight mistruth on the application is, of course!, the weight. The form said "Weight." It did not say "Your current weight." In fact, it did not say "your" weight either, so, in theory, it could have been taken to mean the weight of something unrelated to my own body.

Over a 1.5-ounce serving of chocolate-covered almonds (the healthy dark chocolate), I thought very deeply about this and plodded back to my computer and typed in 140 pounds. Which I have weighed in the not-so-distant past. And I will weigh again in the somewhat-distant future. But at that very moment, when I clicked submit, my weight was closer to about 154, give or take a half pound.

I clicked submit and to my horror a new screen appeared. The screen said "Thank you for your application. We will review it and contact you once we've made our decision."

Oh god, oh god, oh Ganesh or whatever god is available—I have lied on a yoga application. And it isn't cold yoga, it isn't like I can hide those extra 12 pounds under a turtleneck and high-waistline stirrup pants. I'm going to be trotting around in semi-slinky outfits in a giant mirrored room.

I realize I have no choice. I've got to go straight back to celery, first thing Monday morning. Celery and carrots and chicken broth and 1200 calories a day and then I won't be a liar by the time I get there.

Not so fast, says Pudge Monkey.

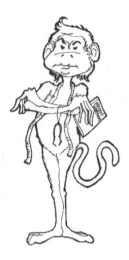

She is having a field day with the slight-mistruth crisis. Pudge Monkey suggests that I have a much bigger problem on hand, one that carrot sticks will never fix. What if my slightly optimistic not-so-current weight of 140 pounds is considered too fat by Mr. Bikram? I mean, at 5'4", the insurance chart says I'm already overweight at 140.

For about a week, I just laid in bed, eyes wide open, like someone with a speed problem only without the colorful cocktail party anecdotes. In the dark, it sometimes seems like if I just concentrate really really hard, it will all make sense, the weight thing.

As always, Prince is so wise. First off, he counsels I get information. Information is all I'm lacking. I e-mail, slightly sheepish, as it has been only nine days, and I ask if I'm in or not and a very nice woman named Shelly writes back six long hours later to say that, yes, I'm in, I've been accepted to Bikram's yoga college.

So, good news, I'm in—bad news is, they are expecting a slightly-less-chubby version of me to show up. Feh. I'll never pull this off.

Again, Prince to the rescue.

"Oh, hon," he coos, his eyes wrinkling like a Shar-Pei.

"It isn't like Bikram is going to stop class and point at you and say 'You are fat!' There will be a sea of people in that room. You are good at blending."

He's right, Prince. I do blend really well. But this seems like quite a tall order. Almost like asking a round Mentos mint to hide amidst a sea of TicTacs.

SATURDAY 22 JANUARY

# of consecutive days doing yoga: 20
# of days until I leave for yoga boot camp: 78

Great day all in all. Got news that we have a buyer for Prince's house. Hoorah! It has been such a long slog—it was a year ago that we mapped out how to finish the tear-out. Also, it was six months ago that I knew I just could not live in that house. Too far away from everything, for starters. Not really my style of a house. Plus which, no yoga studio for nearly 20 miles. We had initially thought we'd slap some paint on the outside and call it a day. But then once you get started, it's like potato chips: you can't just have one. Once the outside looked good, then the inside looked a little dingy.

Our agent convinced us to price the house low, low, low so we could percolate a bidding war. How fun!

A week into it, after getting stupid low-ball offers, people wanting us to take an additional 10 percent off our already-underpriced home—we yanked the listing. The agent said it wasn't what was done. But the final straw for me was when he laughed and said, "But, listen, it is only 12 thousand dollars (less than our asking price). I mean, c'mon, be reasonable, who really gets hung up on 12 grand?"

How silly of me! Twelve thousand dollars is buckets of money. If I did choose to casually toss 12 grand around, that would mean no pedicures for fourteen years.

But then, why should I alone suffer? I could spread out the pain a little and say no pedicures for seven years, no poodle grooming for seven years.

Yeesh.

I talked to mum. She's quite skilled at throwing me off the scent when I'm all het up. She said that in order to sell the house, we needed to buy a Saint Joseph statue. She said it even works on Lutherans—he's a multi-denominational saint. Great website—www.stjosephstatue.com--solved the problem of where to find a saint. We put him in the ground, upside down, one week ago—and one week later, Mr.12Grand became sickly, we got a new agent, and now the phone is jangling.

Just when I didn't think the day could get any better—we passed a street fair on the way back into the city. Big giant banner flapping in the wind: "Wheat-Free Bread."

Yum. How exciting.

Prince cuts across three lanes of traffic and scores an excellent parking space. The bread is made from some until-recently obsolete grain called emmer. Never heard of it before. The sales guy Ryan hands me a handful of the grain, roasted and salted. I'm leery. I quiz him about his claim of wheat-free bread, I ask about what else he bakes in his bakery. He seems incredibly knowledgeable and I'm almost feeling like a fool for not having heard of this magic emmer. Still mulling the salted grain in my hand, Ryan says the magic words: "This is the perfect bread for celiacs."

(Celiac being the medical term for those of us essentially allergic to wheat, barley, oats and rye. Technically, I'm intolerant of those grains. But I think intolerance implies choice. For example, I am intolerant of Naugahyde shoes and the Ku Klux Klan. I digress...)

Hoorah! He knows the right word. Some people think that being wheat-free is a lifestyle choice, like Atkins or kosher. But when the celiac word gets bandied about, then I know I'm in good hands.

I chomp on the emmer grain bits and it is like nothing I have ever tasted.

I decide to delay my bread gratification. Prince and I have a yoga class to get to.

We bought butternut squash soup for dinner. We plan our entire meal around the delish bread. Can't wait to call Frannie and Susan (my wheat-free friends) and tell them of my great find.

MONDAY 24 JANUARY

# of consecutive days doing yoga: 22
# of days until yoga boot camp: 76
# of emmer-induced pimples: 7

The bread was phenomenal—and filled with wheat. We decide, first, to overdress the salad so we can mop up the dressing with the bread, and about 20 minutes into it, I'm dog, dog sick. Most of the awfulness was over in less than four hours—but all night long, horrendous abdominal pain, beet-red ringing ears, a few minor seizures, the whole shooting match. By noon on Sunday, I had sprouted seven new white puss-filled pimples.

I called the bakery and left a message.

Then, hopped online and quickly discovered that emmer is simply another word for wheat. I cannot fathom why the guy would lie. I keep thinking maybe it is the flu that just happened to begin the minute I put their bread in my mouth. But no. Emmer is wheat, no two ways around it.

I sent them an e-mail as well. Hopefully, they'll offer to at least refund the $18 we spent on their bread ($9 a loaf and they lie—the nerve!) and, at the bare minimum, apologize for putting my health in jeopardy.

SUNDAY 30 JANUARY

# of consecutive days doing yoga: 28
# of days until yoga boot camp: 70
# of emmer-induced pimples: 11

Somehow, through the haze of emmer-induced illness, I mucked my way through this past week. I've now got 11 white pussy pimples down the side of my face and I caught a cold—the wheat KOs my immune system. And clumps of hair have fallen out. I'm almost embarrassed to go to the yoga studio. By summer time, they'll be my employer and I'm not exactly looking like a shining example of health.

However—today is day #28 of my 90-day challenge. Hoorah! That's the good news.

However, as I'm ticking off each day of my challenge, simultaneously, I'm that much closer to the beginning of yoga school. It's now under the 3-month mark, which slightly makes my heart thump.

You can't just buy a space heater, hang out a shingle, and teach Bikram Yoga. You've got to attend his intensive nine-week training. And, you have to get approval directly from Bikram.

Bikram wrote a script explaining how to do each posture in the 90-minute class. All teachers must use the script. The script is referred to as simply "the Dialogue." You've got to memorize the Dialogue word-for-word in order to graduate. And, more pressing, you have to deliver the first five minutes of the Dialogue in front of Bikram. Each and every student stands up and recites the words back to the man who authored them.

As I munch on celery sticks and try to visualize thinner thighs, I'm also devoting four hours a day to studying. In addition to memorizing the Dialogue, I'm reading an anatomy book that was written specifically for yoga teachers. I want my brain stuffed as full as possible before I arrive. I think it's the only way I'll survive.

However, with less than 70 days until school, I've barely committed one page of Dialogue to memory. There are 41 pages of Dialogue. It doesn't take a fancy calculator to see that I've got to pick up the pace. Somehow. I started taking Ginkgo biloba, hoping that will help.

I tell Frankie (one of the studio owners) I'm a little wigged out about memorizing the Dialogue. She offers to meet with me every two weeks and she'll pretend to be my student and I'll recite what I've learned. I like having a game plan.

Frankie said that Bikram is tough but also really funny. Laura (the other owner of the studio) heartily agreed. I felt silly, since both Frankie and Laura seem very zenny and at-peace-ish—but I confessed I'm worried that I'm not exactly very bendy. And I'm definitely too round. It seems like if I were bendy then that would make up for my wobble thighs. And vice versa, if I were built like a praying mantis, then my inflexibility wouldn't be such a big deal. I keep thinking of my little round Mentos body surrounded by TicTacs.

Anyhoo, both Frankie and Laura assure me that there will be zero one-on-one corrections. That, honestly, he's teaching 250 students in a big giant room. Only the lucky (and usually the bendy) ones get chosen to have one-on-one corrections from Bikram.

I sleep better, knowing that he's eyes-off and hands-off.

Though I do have a long list of questions for him. For example, in Awkward Pose, he promises: "For you ladies... who have a few pounds of surplus cottage cheese hanging about... this pose is it." I'm still not seeing that happen, even after 28 days. So what's up with that?

Got on the scales today. 157. Damnit damnit damnit. It feels like the nanosecond I started chopping veggies for lunch, my body decided to do a U-turn and rebel. This is totally unfair. Especially with doing yoga every day.

TUESDAY 1 FEBRUARY

# of consecutive days doing yoga: 30
# of days until yoga boot camp: 68
# of emmer-induced pimples: 14

I had this nightmare, woke me up out of a dead sleep, drenched in sweat.

It won't take a fancy dream analyzer to see that I'm struggling with my alleged "authority figure issue"—and facing this head-on with Mr. MyBallsWeighTwoTons Bikram.

I'm replaying one of my first authority encounters. I'm eight and there's a boy, Brian, who keeps picking on me. Shoving me. I had asked the recess monitor about the shoving and she said, "Boys always do that when they like girls." I show her my bruised shins and she smiles a sugary smile and says that I must bruise easily, like I'm daft for not seeing through this whole its-okay-to-be-kicked thing.

Two days after the shin-bruising discussion with the recess monitor, Brian the bully confronts me and starts to kick me and I say (somewhat cockily, as I recall—I thought I had some inside track on how adults operated), "The recess monitor said you kick me because you like me."

Brian the bully replied with, "Oh, yeah. Well, I must really like you a lot today." With that, he kicks me right in between the legs. It was my first experience with both a mean-spirited sociopath and white-hot searing pain.

It was also my first glimpse at a genuine conspiracy cover up.

I limp up to the recess monitor and I point between my legs and I'm crying and I say, "What does it mean if a boy kicks you down there?" And she's looking at me funny—she was watching it from afar, I'm quite sure of it. And she says in a hushy tone, "Sometimes boys don't know their own strength. You'll be fine. Now—go on—go play. Make some new friends."

And I'm thinking, oh, no, I've been kicked down there, I am not currently in a friend-making kind of mood. I asked her, "Who owns the school?" And she blinked funny and asked what I meant, did I mean the principal?

I said thank you and turned on my heel and marched myself to the principal's office.

The secretary outside the principal's office was, I thought, quite snotty at first. She said, "Only parents get to see the principal. He's too busy for little girls."

So I whisper, "A boy kicked me down there." I point down, for effect.

I'm wearing a skirt, so she sees the bruises on my shins and titters a little and says, "That boy must like you then!"

I'm not certain why adults think it is okay for boys to hit girls, but down there really hurts and I'm pretty certain that's an important area and so I stress, again, whispering loudly, "No, down there."

Still no luck, she barely looks up from the typewriter and she ruffles my bangs and says, "Better get back to recess before the bell rings."

"He kicked me right in the vagina."

I'm mortified at saying that word out loud, but something had to be done. Suddenly, like in those old E. F. Hutton commercials, all the heads turn and everyone is looking at me and I'm thinking, oh, dear, I must have said it wrong. I looked it up in the encyclopedia once but the encyclopedia did not say how to say it out loud. I did say vah-jye-nah. But chances are, based on the looks I'm getting, I'm thinking maybe vah-gee-nah would have been better. I also think I said it kind of loudly as it hurt and I didn't want my head patted any more.

I take advantage of the frozen secretaries and I march up to the corner office (assuming that the owner of the school would have the nicest place)—and I open the door and I say to the man behind the desk, "A boy named Brian kicked me in the vagina and it hurts and I don't want it to happen again and your recess monitor should be fired. Also, there's blood and I'll need a nurse, please."

The man behind the desk buzzed the intercom for a nurse and as I was being led away, I heard him say, "Get her parents in here."

He sounded quite terse and angry and, at that time, even then, I haven't even had a decade on the planet and I smelled this whiff of sexism. Like it was less egregious for girls to be kicked down there than boys. Like if the roles were reversed, and I had kicked Brian the bully down there, that the principal would have a much different course of action.

The principal also gave me the impression that I was in trouble, which made me mad, because shouldn't the kicker's parents be phoned as well?

As it unfolded later, my parents said there was concern at the school that I had used the word vagina. They were unable to explain why vagina was a bad word. It was in the encyclopedia and I don't think the encyclopedia would put bad words in their nice leather books. Nonetheless, I was secretly quite pleased to know that I had pronounced it correctly.

Anyway, in my nightmare, everything is unfolding as it happened three decades ago. Kick, recess monitor, snotty secretary. I march down the hallway to the corner office. When I open the door, I'm amazed by the sparkling opulence of the room. It glitters. There are Hindu chotchkes and incense and the desk is kind of a smoky brown glass. Behind the desk is Bikram.

His eyes are sparkly and bright in a supernatural way. I don't want to look into the eyes, they seem snake-ish, as though they will simply hypnotize you into submission.

He smiles a sly, wry smile, almost as though he can't believe I haven't noticed that it has been him all along behind the desk.

He says, "Hello. Why are you here?"

And I am mute, I simply cannot remember why I am there.

Then I wake up, drenched in sweat, heart pounding.

WEDNESDAY 2 FEBRUARY

# of consecutive days doing yoga: 31
# of days until yoga boot camp: 67
# of emmer-induced pimples: 16.5

My first meeting with Frankie went well this morning. I don't know why, but I thought we'd just sit on the floor and I'd recite what I've learned and then we'd be done with it.

I took the noon class and then we went back into the studio after all the students were gone. Frankie put down a mat and was my "student" while I "taught" her using the Dialogue I had memorized (Half Moon and the first two parts of Awkward).

Frankie explained that this is what we will do in yoga college. A few folks will get up on mats and be the students while the teacher-in-training recites the Dialogue. Even if the Dialogue is said incorrectly, the student does exactly as instructed.

I've spent years in front of a live audience, scads of radio and smatterings of live television. In my spare time, I have put a lot of improvisational comedy under my belt. So I wasn't really worried about my presentation skills.

Yet nothing prepared me for this. I was utterly nervous. It might have been a new flu, but I do think it was nerves. My face was flushed and my stomach felt like it was popping kernels of corn and my palms were sweaty. I got mixed up and said left when I meant right and vice versa and all of a sudden Frankie was twisted in a very bad way.

So I said, "Um, okay. Frankie. Okay. I get it. I know, I screwed up. Just fix, you know, what you need to fix."

And she said, "I'm sorry, this is my first Bikram Yoga class and I don't know how to fix things. I'm just doing what you told me to do. You are the teacher."

It dawned on me: I could maim people. And that made me sweat more, and then the popcorn in my stomach felt like sloshy spinach and sour milk and then I had a new revelation. Pity the shy! Until this afternoon, I hadn't a clue how anyone could be timid. In fact, I used to think that shy people had simply run out of good conversational tidbits. But to sweat and stammer and feel sick like this—if this is what shy feels like, oh god, those poor tortured souls.

Frankie said she was impressed with what I had memorized—but also cautioned that I needed to say the words verbatim. Sigh. I was afraid of that. Some of the phrases are just plain wrong. I have even thought of writing to Bikram and asking if he would like me to edit the Dialogue a little bit.

For example, in Half Moon, the body tends to twist a little bit and you want everything in one line. So I'm supposed to say, "right shoulder forward, opening your chest like a flower petal blooming."

Who would say that? First off, the flower petal doesn't do the blooming, per se. The flower does bloom and open, but the single petal doesn't bloom and who would talk like that?

In Hands to Feet, as the teacher is encouraging everyone to try and lock their knees, the Dialogue says that you are creating a tremendous stretch bones to skin, coccyx to toes. That sounds great, doesn't it? Then, "coccyx to the toes with your smiling happy face."

Who would say that? I mean, maybe, maybe if I were trying to calm a colicky baby, I might maybe utter something like "smiling happy face." Plus which, it is a run-on sentence. Plus which, it just doesn't make sense.

In the first part of Awkward Pose, with the students stretching their arms straight out in front of them, the Dialogue says, "triceps nice and tight, contraction."

That's just plain grammatically wrong. And, as a writer and an English major, I can't do bad grammar. I simply can't.

So I figured I'd slightly edit those things when I was saying the Dialogue in front of Frankie.

She noticed! I don't know why that surprised me either, I figured that the Dialogue is sort of like when I had the TelePrompTer in front of me in my broadcasting days: a slush pile of good ideas hiding behind poorly-organized words, there for my use, to break open in case of emergency.

Not that Bikram isn't a yoga guru, I don't doubt that. But English is his second language, so it makes sense that the Dialogue would sound like that—someone struggling with a new language.

I told Frankie I'd be glad to help Bikram edit the Dialogue a bit. She laughed and rolled her eyes a bit and said I had to memorize and say the words exactly as they are written in the Dialogue.

(I do wonder, though, if Bikram has some kind of brainwashing built into the training. It seems hard to imagine that a normal sane grown adult would embrace these words without any kind of questioning.)

Nonetheless, I'll meet with Frankie in two more weeks—she's asked me to memorize all the way through Standing Head to Knee, the fifth posture.

I ask Frankie, again, about Bikram. What's he like up close and in person?

She said he's funny and he's quite sure of himself. He proclaims he is the "Prince of Beverly Hills." She thinks he might be stubborn. She said the most important thing to remember is that he views his studio in Los Angeles as his home and he is protective of it.

And don't wear green—I remember that, right?

I ask about 67 questions about the no-green rule. It is just plain weird. Plus there's no reason to it—why no green? Besides, he can't possibly hate green--trees are green and grass is green and sometimes the ocean turns aqua green. Speaking of aqua, what shades of green? There are so so so many greens. Mint and aqua and olive and kelly and hunter and forest and grass and pea soup and lime and sage.

What about that green unitard I just bought? I can't wear it?

What about money, money is green, and he happily takes my money, right, so isn't that a tacit acceptance of green?

Frankie listens patiently, though I think her eyes have the glassy look of disinterest. She asks me if I have "authority figure issues."

I think of kindergarten lunch and the third grade recess conspiracy and the fifth grade social studies guy and the eleventh grade band director and twelfth grade driver's education dude and freshman college band director (gawd, that was a debacle of epic proportions) and sophomore journalism teacher and my first boss in New York City.

I fudge it and reply, "Umm, no, not really."

Maybe this is the union of mind and body that yoga always talks about. My mind wants to reject smarty-pants egomaniacs but my body will learn to shush.

I vow, on this day, I will keep my eyes down like an obedient geisha, I will say nothing, I will not even look him in the eyes.

FRIDAY 11 FEBRUARY

# of consecutive days doing yoga: 40
# of days until yoga boot camp: 58
# of emmer-induced pimples: 13

When I dropped my freelance jobs to devote myself to yoga-ing full time, I worried I would be bored.

Instead, most days I feel like there aren't enough hours.

Between Dialogue memorization, plodding through the anatomy book, and going to the yoga studio every single day, it seems I'm left with about one "spare" hour.

(Though if you factor ongoing ackiness due to emmer incident and time off to go to the doctor's office and at least 20 minutes each day trying to mentally adjust to all the new acne scars—then I'm at a deficit for sure.)

Whatever spare time I have left is devoted to my quest for affordable housing whilst at yoga boot camp. Most days, this feels like an exercise in utter futility. Bikram's training headquarters are located in Beverly Hills, California. Not exactly a place where "budget" comes to mind. Bikram offers dormitory-style housing—two-bedroom apartments with five students crammed in. Isn't that awful? Plus which, it isn't cheap—$2,100 to be smooshed in with complete strangers.

I've realized that at a certain age, there are some things you just can't or won't or shouldn't do. Paying over 2,000 dollars to sleep on a sofa bed and share a potty with 4 other people— nope, not this chick. I'm convinced I can find something similar, and yet, less crowded, less spendy.

If need be, I will sell some of my fancy television suits on eBay so I can afford a slightly better place to live. It is good to clean out closets, the black is totally depressing, and it is also symbolic. I am shedding old habits, just like my runes told me to.

FRIDAY 18 FEBRUARY

# of consecutive days doing yoga: 47
# of days until yoga boot camp: 51
# of hours w/angry Russian facialist hell bent on restoring skin to
pre-emmer glow: 2.75

Happy anniversary to me and my colon!

Seven years ago today, I was diagnosed with nontropical celiac sprue. When I told a friend of mine the news, she said, "Aw, that's a shame, the sprue." Sounded awful, even, "the sprue."

(Thankfully, over the years, the disease's name has been shortened to celiac.)

I had been sickly for years. Rotating weird stuff. Like my hands would double in size, just puff right up for about six weeks and then I'd wake up one morning and they'd be normal again. My hair would fall out in clumps; my abdomen would bloat until I looked like I was with child. Giant purple pimples everywhere. Seizures, but those had been there a long time. Sinus pain. Irritability. Stabbing bone pain.

No one could ever figure it out. Which makes sense, in a way. When I went to a gastrointestinal specialist, I didn't dwell on the hair falling out or the bone pain. Likewise, when at the neurologist's, I didn't mention my ongoing tummy woes. Different doctors, different body parts.

I did have a naturopathic chiropractor who diagnosed it at my very first appointment with him. He was doing strength testing and said, "How is your digestion? What color are your stools?" My knee-jerk, none-of-your-business reaction was "Fine." I mean, that's creepy, you know? There I am, hoping to get my frozen shoulder thawed with the bone guy and he's asking for vivid description of bowel output.

A few years after the psychic chiropractor, I had minor surgery, and while I was out, the doctor decided to poke around and look for endometriosis. That was sort of the last chance at the OK Corral diagnosis; I had tested negative for everything else under the sun. The surgeon reports that there was not a drop of endometriosis lying around. Not even some old scars lying around. Once again, no explanation for the tummy pain. Damnit.

Perversely, the surgery gave me my answer. Not the answer I expected, but an answer nonetheless.

I got violently ill after the surgery, thought it was the flu. Ten days into it, I'm too sick for my post-op followup. I remember telling the doctor that my entire left side hurt; if he dropped me, that was okay, but I just wanted to know why just my left hand had swollen this time.

The Prior Husband and I have to cancel our Valentine's Day plans—I just can't get off the couch and/or stop rolling around on the cool tile bathroom floor long enough to get dressed and socialize like a regular human.

Oddly, one day later, I suddenly feel well enough to go out. We meet friends, Jeff and Amy, at an Indian restaurant. I do so love their bread, the naan. Even more so when they fill it with garlic and cheesy bits. Anyway, I'm making good headway into the naan basket when suddenly, my left hand swells, my ears feel weird and I excuse myself and try to walk with some sort of nonpanicked dignity to the toilette. Violently ill. Sweaty. Probably the flu. Probably should just go home but The Prior Husband has been (rightfully, I suppose) a little petulant about all my odd, unpredictable symptoms.

Splash my face with water, pinch my cheeks for the healthy rosy look, reapply lip gloss. Walk calmly and confidently back to the dinner table, have some rice, another yummy triangle of garlic naan. Blam. Sweaty, ears ringing, tongue feels fat, slightly less dignity in my mad toilette dash.

Splash, pinch cheeks, gloss lips. Table. Rice. Naan.

I'm embarrassed to even admit this, but on piece of naan number four, our friend Jeff leaned over and whispered, "Why don't you skip the naan?"

"But I love the naan." I feel offended. Who doesn't love cheese-stuffed bread?

"I know. But I think it is making you sick."

I am shocked. What the hell is he talking about? There's a flu going around, it is that season, it is that part of the country. Naan is good, Jeff is bad. I'm slightly miffed, frankly. I've got to talk to The Prior Husband about who we socialize with when we get home.

Jeff presses forward.

"I've just noticed over the past year or so that when we eat here and you eat naan, you tend to excuse yourself and go to the, ah, um, you know, the bathroom and your face looks kind of flushed when you return . . .."

I cut him off. Honestly. Quite cheeky really. I mean, I know he's a veterinarian and all, but talking about potty issues should never ever be done, let alone during dinner in front of other people. Plus which, he's pushed the naan basket out of my reach and I want my naan.

His wife overhears his muted comments and looks a little alarmed.

"You know, Jeff, she does look like she's having an allergic reaction."

His willing conspirator, Jeff's wife slides the naan bread entirely to the other side of the table.

The Prior Husband chuckles and says, "She always looks like that at dinner." He's a jolly one, and, as an only child, has an astonishingly well-honed ability to self amuse. He's chuckling and eating my share of naan; meanwhile, Jeff and Amy seem alarmed at Prior's nonchalance.

Jeff was diagnosed with celiac two decades earlier, during college. Jeff explains that the primary "textbook" symptoms of that disease are severe malnutrition and wretched weight loss. He's 6 feet tall and when he was finally diagnosed, he weighed a scant 84 pounds.

Jeff says that since underweight isn't an issue of mine, I don't have celiac. But probably some other issue. He explains that a doctor will most likely put me on this gluten-free diet for starters, so he advises that I eat boiled chicken and rice and drink Gatorade for the next week or so and see if I get better.

The whole incident was really unsettling. First off, I felt accused of something. Secondly, to have someone move the breadbasket away from you like you are some kind of bread junkie needing salvation—well, who wants that in the middle of a perfectly nice dinner? Thirdly, I felt awfully excluded. Like "You can't have our bread" combined with "You couldn't possibly have my illness because you are too fat to have what I have."

Mostly to prove Jeff wrong, on February 18, 1998, I went to a doctor. Pulled his name out of the yellow pages. I have preferred women doctors in the past, but I was just so sick, I took the first appointment available.

I relay the Indian dinner incident to the doctor and he smiles and gets excited and says, "I know exactly what you have. I'm going to write it down on a piece of paper and slip it in my pocket. I think you know what the problem is too. Keep talking, keep talking! Then, we'll compare notes!"

So we get to the end of the road and he pronounces me celiac. An allergy, of sorts, to wheat, barley, oats, and rye. Says he just loves handing out this diagnosis. Best thing in the world! He hands me a brochure and says, "Do you have any questions?"

"So no donuts?"

(I always treated myself to a Dunkin' Donut on Thursdays, weigh-in day. Plus which, I could see the Dunkin Donuts out the window—right across the street from Dr. NoWheat.)

"No. No donuts. No wheat, barley, oats or rye. Listen, this is a great thing. I love this disease! You'll just have to buy different food at the store. No drugs, no pills, no side effects. Just put down the cookies and pick up the green beans."

Eff you, perky diagnostic boy. Who has ever said, "Mmm. Feeling like a little dessert tonight. I know, I'm really in the mood for fresh hot steaming broccoli"?

I try to appeal to the doctor's logic.

"Yesterday I could eat wheat. So what you are saying is that, magically, today I cannot eat wheat? I mean, at the very least, you owe me a donut. I wasn't going to say anything earlier, but I was going to stop and get a donut before the appointment and I didn't want to be late. So if I had disrespected your busy schedule, I could be sinking my teeth into a sugar-glazed bow tie right about now?"

He smiles nicely. No doubt he's heard this before.

"Just say no. Here's the brochure. There's a good health food store about 20 miles away. Any other questions not related to donuts?"

"So if I had a donut hole, that would be less wheat, right?"

And round and round we went. The very patient Dr. NoWheat worked me through my bargaining phase. No donut holes, no donut holes cut in half, no licking of donut holes.

The first year was utter hell. Food is such an inextricable part of our lives. For about six months, I had this recurring nightmare. I've gone back to college. I'm assigned two perky roommates—the girls from the Triscuit commercials. You know the ones—"Are you are the new girl in town? Hungry? How about a little Triscuit nachos? No? Not your style? Okay. Triscuit and fruit? Triscuit and ranch dressing?"

I march myself to the Dean's office (shades of the third grade principal visit?). The Dean says I have to learn to live with wheat all around me and that it is fun and exciting to be free of wheat. I try to explain that I'm not anti-wheat necessarily, I just don't think I should be forced to live with the Triscuit fan club president.

The Triscuit nightmares eventually ended, and ultimately, I eat so well now, so healthy. I've settled into my funky little gluten-free routine—though, admittedly, yoga boot camp will put that to the test. It's probably the biggest reason I'm trying (desperately, I might add) to find my own little roommate-free haven while yoga-ing for nine weeks.

First off, there's the contamination issue. If someone puts butter on their toast and the toast crumbs get left on the butter—I'm dog sick.

Taking it a step further, even breadcrumbs left on a toaster have slayed me—so I have bought my own toaster for the trip. (Which I'm not complaining—it was an excellent excuse to buy the long-coveted Hello Kitty toaster, which toasts Kitty's face on the bread!)

In all honesty, convenience issues aside, the worst thing about being celiac is trying to explain all this to food allergy virgins. If they've never in their life been exposed to any kind of food allergy, they just think you are a little overly compulsive. Plus which, with Atkins and other low-carb diets booming, a lot of people think that wheat/gluten-free is a dietary choice and that it wouldn't kill me if a small bit of soy sauce (which is, viciously, distilled with wheat) is splashed on my asparagus.

(Some day, when I run into extra money, I will make soy sauce my hobby. It shouldn't be labeled soy sauce since it has wheat in it. I've even seen some brands of "soy sauce" {finger quotes heavily used here} that don't even have any soy in them. Just wheat, water, and salt as ingredients. Totally unfair and deceptive and false advertising and what have you.)

So how can I possibly think that four other roommates would get it? And how can I share a fridge with all those people? I need space, lots of space. Plus which, I totally want this experience to be as yummy as humanly possible. Aside from the divorce, this is my first big capital-intensive investment in myself. I cannot put it in jeopardy.

FRIDAY 25 FEBRUARY

# of consecutive days doing yoga: 54
# of days until yoga boot camp: 44

Found a roommate. Actually, a week ago I had agreed to room with this girl named Yok (pronounced like egg yolk). About 12 hours later, another gal surfaced and then I had two roommates and then I was totally confused, how could I pick?

I proposed that all three of us share a place and spent most of last week trying to find something that would easily accommodate three of us without beginning to feel like a dorm again.

Yok is from Thailand and very sweet and replies to my e-mails pretty quickly. Seems like she might be shy and quiet, though. She's married to a tall Nordic man. Cannot fathom how they met.

Jessica is the other end of the rainbow: loud and funny and from New Jersey with big pouffy hair and a great laugh. She described her dream job as "flamenco dancer."

I had been spending the bulk of my time pawing through www.craigslist.com, looking at the rental section for Los Angeles. It seemed like each and every ad on the website was posted by a flake, a snot, or a psychopath. I'd find a great place, only to get to the lease signing and find out that they wanted the rent paid in full at the beginning in cash. Or that they'd want three months' rent despite the fact we'll be there for two months. Or, my personal favorite, they wanted to meet in person to see if you'd be "right" for their rental unit.

Right when I was on the cusp of giving a deposit on a house that would be great for three of us, Jessica wrote to say she had found a great place within walking distance of the school. Bah. A little sad—but relieved. Still not sure where Yok and I are going to live, but finding a place for two will be easier in the long run.

Had another fake class with Frankie today. I got all the way through the first 30 minutes of class. Frankie still stressing that I recite the Dialogue verbatim. She's really noticing the parts that I've, shall we say, enhanced with better language.

In posture #5, Standing Head to Knee, the Dialogue is addressing having a locked knee, and the fourth sentence reads, "You don't have the knee."

I said it a smidge differently, saying that your leg is so locked out that "you no longer have a kneecap, it is now invisible." Which isn't that far from "You don't have the knee." Still, Frankie stressed the importance of saying it as it is printed on the page.

I asked if it was the kind of thing where I say it his way when he's around and then when I graduate, I use some of what I think works and she said no. Color me surprised. She also said that I'll be an apprentice with her for the first six months after graduation, and she'll expect me to say it verbatim for those first six months.

Frankie also said I need to start moving my mat to different parts of the room when I come in to practice. She said something about yoga being a practice in detachment.

(I bit my tongue; I wanted so madly to quip, "Actually, by reciting Bikram's dorky words, I'm practicing detachment from the English language." I love being wise! I know I would have said that if I were in my 30s.)

She also reminded me that there are quite a few studios in the area and that I should practice at other studios before I go to training.

I was telling Frankie of my roommate travails. She said the important thing to keep in mind is that I'll make friends for a lifetime. On the way home, I think that the friends thing would be nice. I've had so many mentally challenged friends (the one who tried to light my wedding dress on fire, por ejemplo)—once I realized I needed sane people in my life, my datebook got a little bare.

4 MARCH

# of consecutive days doing yoga: 61
# of days until yoga boot camp: 37

I called the Bikram's Yoga College of India headquarters today. Very odd little world.

Our money was due in full by March 1. I sent in my check a few weeks ago and it hasn't ever been cashed. Now that I've memorized parts of the Dialogue and found a roommate, the last thing I'd want to happen is getting ejected from school before I get there.

Spoke to an exotic-sounding person. Not even sure if it was a man or a woman. Just a name that sounded like an Indian dinner special and a husky, lilting voice. The voice said, "Dear, we don't have time to go to the bank every day. We have enough money to tie us over without your check."

I thought it was kind of snotty-sounding and was a bit taken aback by it, but I suppose the voice had a good point. I tried to explain my reasoning—I just didn't want to get kicked out.

The voice laughed a genuine laugh and said, "Once you are in, you are in for good."

I think that sounds a little cult-ish.

Had that same dream again last night—the walking to the principal's office, opening the door, opulence and glitter everywhere, Bikram behind the desk.

"Why are you here?"

It is interesting, he doesn't sound angry or accusatory—just a simple statement. I still don't want to look into his eyes.

And I don't know that I have the answer to his question. Why am I doing this? I was hoping my thighs would shape up with his allegedly miraculous yoga and that hasn't happened yet. So I'd like to ask him that. And I thought yoga was about inner peace, but my mind monkeys are still nagging me.

11 MARCH 2005

# of consecutive days doing yoga: 68
# of days until yoga boot camp: 30

Taught another fake class with Frankie as my student. Got all the way through Balancing Stick, posture #7. She's put me on the schedule to teach a real class before I leave—which, oh Ganesh, is now right at 30 days. I had so wanted to have the whole Dialogue memorized and each line feels like a struggle to get it to stay in my brain.

I tried writing it out longhand, but that didn't work so well. Then I tried typing it over and over and that worked about 10 percent of the time. The rest of the time I was struggling with not rewriting the thing. Frankie says the only way to do it is to say the Dialogue out loud over and over again.

She also asked, again, if I've been going to other studios to practice. I like my studio—and I do like my spot under the heater. Frankie again says it is best that I learn to detach.

(Part of me is beginning to wonder—is Frankie getting too attached to pushing me into detachment?)

15 MARCH 2005

# of consecutive days doing yoga: 72
# of days until yoga boot camp: 26

I really am starting to like the early morning 6:45 class. Laura usually teaches the early class and I like her style. She's had her first baby and lots of times talks about what she's learning from motherhood and I look forward to hearing those stories.

After class today, she asked me if I had gone to another studio yet. Sometimes I wonder—maybe there's some hidden reason to get me to go elsewhere?

Laura also said I need to move my mat to a different spot. That it is good to not be attached to any one area.

(What is it with these yoga people? What the hell is wrong with a little attachment anyway?)

Frankie had said that it would be pretty crowded at training and Laura stressed that this morning as well.

Laura said when she was at yoga boot camp, "Some students would roll up like water bugs and run to put their mat in the good spots. But that's no way to make friends. And you are so social, just enjoy the entire experience and don't worry about where your mat ends up."

I know I was supposed to take home a zen-ish spots-don't-matter message from Laura's wisdom. But the message that pinged into my brain like a heat-seeking missile was: there are good spots to be had at yoga boot camp.

I asked her to clarify, where exactly were the good spots?

Laura laughed and said something about me being funny. She also she said she just knew that I wouldn't be the type to get hung up on finding a good spot.

I feel thwarted, damnit. She knows something that I need to know.

18 MARCH

# of consecutive days doing yoga: 75
# of days until yoga boot camp: 23

Mostly to get Frankie off my back, I went to practice at a studio over on the eastside, out to the 'burbs.

I give it a positive spin and decide that a new studio means I can meet new teachers this way and learn new tricks about surviving yoga boot camp.

First off, there was no friendly greeting upon my arrival, like there is at the Sweatbox. The Sweatbox feels like Cheers to me. You walk in, everyone knows your name. The teacher was incredibly detached. I introduced myself and the teacher, Tili, doesn't even look up from the keyboard. No eye contact.

I congratulated her and said that she was teaching the seventy-fifth day of my 90-day challenge and she shrugged. Shrugged! Seventy-five consecutive days of yoga is not something to shrug at, literally or figuratively. I should have just left right then and there. Why should I detach when she can't detach? It isn't fair, really, when you get down to it.

The studio was stupidly wicked hot. There were three dozen students and it was so hot that by the half-way point, over one dozen were laying on the floor panting. With 15 minutes left in class, only 3 of us were left standing.

After class, Tili made a snotty comment about how the Sweatbox could never attract a good crowd, not without showers. I'm shocked speechless. I just sort of thought all the teachers would be nice like Frankie and Laura.

She was curious, though, as to how her class compared to the Sweatbox. I said something about her class being a lot drippier than what I'm used to. I asked when she graduated from yoga boot camp—three years ago. I told her I was going—did she know if there was a good spot in the room?

"Oh, definitely. On the right hand side of the room, towards the center."

I'm a-titter with excitement. I'm honing in on that answer which I do desperately seek.

"Which side though? The right side if you are standing in the back facing the front of the room? Or standing front, facing back?"

She looked at me with raw contempt and repeated what she said. "The good spots are on the right side of the room."

As if to underscore my idiocy, she rolls her eyes dramatically.

What is with these people withholding valuable information from me? It is just wrong. And seems very un-yogic, right? Isn't yoga the union of body and mind? So my body needs to know what is in her mind—what the hell is wrong with that?

Then Tili hits me with the zinger. "If I were you, I'd reconsider training. The heat here in this studio is about one-tenth the heat Bikram likes during training. Finding the right spot won't fix anything if you are already weak to begin with."

I am wounded and beyond concealing my hurt.

She smiles a nice vixen smirky smile and pats me on the arm and says, "That's okay, hon. I think you can still get your deposit back."

What a mean, mean person. Isn't that awful? Telling me to get my money back! She didn't even say the Dialogue. I should ask her for a refund of her class. Wonder if I can turn her in to someone? Maybe there's a toll free number. Like the bumper stickers on trucks that read, "How's my driving?"

Instead, it should be, "How's my teaching? Call 1-800-BAD-YOGA."

Weirdly, though, as I left the studio, the mean-spirited teacher stopped me.

"Do you think you'll really go?"

Good golly, yes. C'mon Tili, you don't honestly think I'd let someone as goofy as you completely alter my life's path, do you?

"You know, enjoy it. You will have a great time and you'll make friends that will last you a lifetime."

Funny. Frankie said the same thing, friends for life. I hope they are both right. New friends would be kind of kicky. I just hope they are nicer than Tili.

19 MARCH 2005

# of consecutive days doing yoga: 76
# of days until yoga boot camp: 22

Today, I woke up, and I thought to myself, "Eff the yoga."

Isn't that awful?

But seriously—75 consecutive days is enough yoga for now. Right? I mean, who else is doing yoga every single day? And what's with the 90-day goal?

Shopping Monkey and Money Monkey were, oddly, in agreement. If I took the next two weeks off and banged out a quick freelance article or two, I'd have extra money to apply to the current quest for thigh-improving yoga shorts.

Pudge Monkey sent in an absentee ballot; she's overly fatigued lately. Standing in front of a mirror every single day has given her a sensory overload. The number of flaws she can point to is often overwhelming and it makes her head spin.

Morality Monkey dissented, pointing out the importance of setting goals and sticking to them.

Glad I went, though. Had a good posture breakthrough.

The fifth posture, Standing Head to Knee, has four distinct parts of the posture.

First, you shift your weight to your left leg and then pick your right foot up in front of you. Keeping that left leg locked, the second part of the posture is kicking the right heel out so that your two legs look like a right angle. Third part is bending your elbows down towards the ground and the last part is putting your forehead on your knee.

Anyway, I just don't ever kick that heel out. I'm not like that, I'm not that kind of gal. Frankie was teaching and she said something along those lines—that if you are in the habit of not kicking out, try it. That's why it is called a yoga practice.

Practice. Of course! I'm not on some stage, I'm practicing.

So—I kicked out. I waited until the second set, though, to make sure everything was just right. And the kick lasted about three and a half seconds. Nonetheless, I can check off that box.

30 MARCH

# of consecutive days doing yoga: 87
# of days until yoga boot camp: 11

As I scuttle around getting ready for this adventure, I keep having flashbacks to two years ago. I did not know it at the time, but I was only a few weeks away from getting the court to stamp my divorce papers and make it all official.

All I knew was that I had to leave. I had served him with papers that previous summer. I believed my attorney down to the pompoms on my socks when she promised that the process would be "quick and easy. We'll have you finalized in four months, six months at the most."

Partially because I believed in the false promise and partially because my Scottish genes prohibit money misuse, the Prior Husband and I continued to live together as we went through the divorcing maze.

Prior Husband really wanted to go to trial. He claimed he wanted his day in court, so he could explain his side of things. Truthfully, though, I think he enjoyed all those silent services I continued to provide: I did laundry, walked the dogs, and maintained our 300-year-old haunted farmhouse. If I left, who would restart the hot water heater or scrub the cat pee off the electrical outlet?

I consulted the Runes and they shouted, "move." Well, shout is a strong word for Runes. But the Foundation tile was the Journey Rune and the Outcome tile was Strength reversed—which always points to new beginnings. For at least a year, I also kept getting the Gateway Rune—that's the one that talks about standing on the hilltop of your life looking down behind you, and the only way you can continue your journey is to bless all that you have had thus far.

Anyway, the Runes told me to leave, which sounds loopy if you haven't ever used Runes.

But at that time, the Runes were the only thing I could count on.

My entire life was hanging in the balance, stalled by one legal delay after another. The Prior Husband was battling chronic depression and I so longed to be surrounded by happy people.

We were estranged in the very fullest sense of the word; I so longed for intimacy I could taste its succor underneath my fingernails.

My frustration at the lack of control of my destiny burbled over into odd projects. For example, I imagined I would just drive away one day, Atlantic to Pacific. I imagined pulling over at a rest stop, firing up the laptop, and e-mailing my board of directors.

(Board of directors is my term for my closest, sweetest friends, the ones I turn to when confused. The true blue friends who will say, "yes, those jeans do, indeed, make your butt look fat.")

Anyway, the problem with my blog plan was I had a four-year-old laptop and a two-year-old cell phone. And the laptop was a Mac. I spent hours on eBay looking for the right cord to connect the phone and the iBook, and then when I got the cord, I needed software for the cord (who knew?)—in the end, weeks later, I cried uncle.

Two years later, the laptop is that much more antiquated, and for about a day I consider buying a used laptop and spending some time bringing the used one up to speed. But then I remembered how hard it was to find the software for the cord. (Cords should not need software. If I had time, I'd write to my Senator about this.)

Anyway, Prince and I went to the Mac store and I indulged in a brand-new laptop. I do know I will lose little bits of sanity if I can't e-mail my board of directors during this new adventure.

Once I addressed my pressing technological needs, I filled the time void with a brand-new project.

I got this great card from mum in the mail. The front of the card reads: "At every crossroad, follow your dream. It is courageous to let your heart lead the way."

On the inside, mum wrote: "This is a perfect calling for you—your students will love you! In my yoga class today, I could picture you teaching—your smile, those sparkling eyes, and your sense of humor winning everyone over."

I sat and cried big fat tears reading that. In some ways, yoga boot camp is mum's handiwork. For years she has called me her "little Dharma." Mum was a big fan of the Dharma & Greg television show. I finally made time to sit down and watch the show, to figure out why she was calling me after the character. At first, I was offended. The Dharma woman is blonde and ditzy and doesn't have a regular job. She helps a Native American carry out his death ritual in their apartment and drives to Reno for pie.

No matter the situation, though, she was always kind. A little goofy, sure. Really cute clothes and pajamas. (Shopping Monkey was most pleased when she found a website dedicated to great sleep wear "as seen on TV." www.sleepwear.tv)

In addition to being kind, Dharma was unwaveringly truthful. Por ejemplo, she didn't put on a serious dark suit and slick her hair back and pretend to be something she's not.

Over time, I loved that mum saw my Dharma potential.

(Interesting side note. Dharma is a Sanskrit word that is often considered tough to translate. Loosely, though, "dharma" means the right way of living, the path of righteousness, justice, doing good.)

After nearly 90 days of yoga, I feel like my postures are okay.

(Actually, I'm most proud of my Rabbit Pose. I always get compliments on it.)

Not necessarily great or anything, but not too shabby. However, that snotty yoga teacher's warning about the heat does haunt me from time to time. I decide I'll need mid-class pep talks, little trinkets or reminders that everything is just like it is at home, only slightly different. I'll make an iron-on decal of inspirational sayings—including my mum's card—for my yoga mat. Got great transfer paper at the craft store—just put it in the printer, print, iron, voila! A personalized, perky yoga mat.

I'm thinking this will take maybe an hour, two hours tops.

First off, my color printer is acting funny. Likes to print in many hues of purple but won't give me orange. Bah. Go to a website and download a thingy for printers with purple-itis. Nothing.

Fine. Breathe. When I'm baking in eight zillion degrees, will I look down and see my mum's words cheering me and think, "Damn, I'd feel cooler if those words were in orange?" Not likely.

When I switch to orange, the printer gives me a sickly regurgitated yellow. Not feeling the perk in that.

I bail on the color altogether and put the transfer paper into the laser printer. And, kerflooey!—the transfer paper is jammed beyond all recognition in the printer. I pop open the laser printer and, oh, okay, perfect sense, of course! The iron-on decal won't budge. It has melted into a smelly lump in the middle of the printer.

My fix-it engineer Prince tries to get the iron-on lump to budge. And Prince has already had a busy day. I declared today Craft Day—getting done noncrucial fun crafty things for the trip. Found a great pink laptop carrying case. My talented Prince easily inked a Hello Kitty on the pink case.

He astonishes me, my Prince. I mean, if I were in a hostage situation and the only way to get the guard to release us was to sketch something, I might pull off a sketch of a stick-figure dog. Maybe. But under normal nonhostage circumstances, drawing is just not in my talent portfolio.

SATURDAY 2 APRIL

# of consecutive days doing yoga: 90
# of days until yoga boot camp: 8

I may not be able to draw. But showing up is a well-honed skill of mine. Today is day #90. Woohoo! I did it. I really truly managed to go to yoga class every single day for 90 consecutive days. I didn't even "cheat" and skip a day or two and then do three classes in a row to make up for it. Nope. Even with the emmer/wheat-induced illness, I came to class.

The results are pretty astonishing.

In 90 days, I have lost one inch in each thigh. Each thigh!! Hips are one inch slimmer. Waist is one inch slimmer. Bust is two inches smaller. And—saving the best for last—I am now one-and-a-half inches taller. Which technically means that at this whopping 5'6" towering height, I am no longer overweight.

Which also means that if I get to Bikramland and someone says, "Wait a minute, you look like you weigh more than you said on your application," I can easily say, "Well, yes. But I grew over two inches."

Can you imagine how lithe I'll be after teacher training? Twice a day—I might be mistaken for an actual thin person by the time this is over.

4 APRIL

of days until yoga boot camp: 6

Against better judgment, Prince and I go to look at a house. We've already been outbid on three houses thus far. Awfully disheartening, really. We both have great credit ratings, he's had the same job for about 70 years, and we both have equity from our Prior Spouses. And yet, we can barely afford a one-bedroom condo the way things are going. However, we really like this house, it has that unique feel we both like and sweet Prince has offered to do all the moving while I'm away.

We've named this house The Fishbowl.

I have named all the houses we've looked at and seriously considered—makes conversations so much easier. Instead of, "You know, Hon, remember that one house on that street and the house had that funny smell and the cross street was Cherry, you know that one?"

"Well, the funny mold smell or the funny cat pee smell?"

"I don't know, Hon, it was just really stinky. That one."

"But there were two houses that were close to Cherry Street. And both were malodorous, but one had shag carpeting."

And so on. At least twice, these which-house chats have escalated to near-arguments.

In the past six months, we have lost out on The Zen House, The Castle, and The Hansel & Gretel House.

We feel good, though, about The Fishbowl. It was built in the early 1970s by Space City Builders—doesn't that sound so Jetsons-y? It has over two-dozen round windows and/or skylights. It has a yummy office area for me with a built-in loft and a wood shop area for Prince. The Realtor tells us that most people are turned off by the round windows. One prior house-shopper said it looked like the house had boils. I think it looks like the house has eyes.

The exterior is a yucky mustard color, so that's easy to fix. Everything else—plumbing, electrical, roof—is in great shape. The owners, we figure, have got to be anxious to sell.

The husband relocated to California; the wife left behind with three children under age six. She's to stay in the house until it sells. Her eyes are a bit wide and buggy, she looks like she's nurturing a rousing case of cabin fever. This is great news for us; she must be simply desperate to sell the house to us this instant.

Did all the paperwork and put the bid in on the house around nine tonight. Lined up an inspector for tomorrow afternoon—we are so sure The Fishbowl will be ours. Our agent tells us the inspector being available is a good omen. Usually the inspector is booked for weeks on end, especially in this gaga market.

Then—started the packing-for-yoga fun. The hardest part was getting all the techno goodies ready. Cell phone and battery and charger. iPod and charger and syncher. Laptop and charger. Mouse and charger.

Once all the bits were unplugged and snug in their new pink Hello Kitty carrier—then on to clothing. Frankie and Laura both stressed that whatever amount of clothing I take with me, it will not be enough. I'm convinced I can sneak in a load of laundry in the middle of the week; they are dubious. Actually, I think Frankie was snickering behind her hand when she said, "Sure. Laundry. In the middle of the week."

I managed to get most everything into two suitcases. Why in god's name it takes one suitcase for a week at my mum's and two for nine weeks—don't know. I remain a little suspicious.

It is midnight now—and still no word on whether they have accepted our offer. The Fishbowl has been on the market over a month, so you'd think they'd be dancing a jig. Prince and I both feel, though, that the universe will provide us with the right house. And while The Fishbowl is great, it would be a bit of a schlep for both of us commute-wise.

Speaking of easy commutes, though: The Fishbowl is less than one mile from Prince's Prior Wife. She's a nice lady and everything; I really do like her. But I wonder if moving so close is a good idea? I don't know why it would be a bad idea, but I so treasure this marriage and I want everything to be done ipsy-pipsy-perfect. Put another way: I don't want to be complaining to my friend Karina that our marriage feels strained and then she'll say, "You know, I kind of wondered about that. Didn't you see the study in Oprah's magazine that said over 80 percent of second marriages that live within a two -mile radius of a prior spouse are more likely to divorce?" And then I'd feel stupid, that I hadn't done all my research.

6 APRIL

Somehow, we managed to get all my goodies into Betty the Bug and were on the road pretty much on schedule. I don't know why, but the monkeys returned in full force. Pudge Monkey was banging her chest about the calorie count of a Starbucks chai latte, Money Monkey was running the numbers, reminding me that it would take over two years to pay off the tuition and Shopping Monkey knew we were doomed. She had talked with Pudge and Money Monkeys and they all agreed that 11 pairs of yoga shorts were not enough and that, given the thigh jiggliness, at least 3 more pairs should be purchased before school starts.

Morality Monkey was again forced to withhold his vote. He tried hard, in his soft and calming voice, to remind everyone that yoga is about uniting body and mind. Yoga is not about shopping.

Morality Monkey's proclamation didn't go over well with the rest of the gang, oddly uniting all three. Money Monkey reminded Morality Monkey that yoga provides money and money provides shopping. Shopping Monkey concurred heartily. And Pudge Monkey reminded everyone that proper clothing will always make me look less chubby.

We got a call from our Realtor mid-drive. It appears that we are not going to be "winning" the house at this time. Magically, out of thin air, five other offers appeared after our offer. Really now? I smell a rat. Our hunch—The Fishbowl agent worked the phones. Didn't even tell the owners we had put in a bid. Just called all the other prospects and added steam to the froth and said "bidding war" and then people lost their minds. We don't ever get to know who the other bidders are—I hate the whole closed system of it all. When I worked on a trading desk, when an offer came through, you could see on the screen—how many shares, how much offered, who offered. Now, our housing fate is in the hands of an agent who says, "My name is Kevin, but please call me Skippy, all my friends do." Yick.

We arrive at our hotel 600 miles later, and there was a fax from our agent saying that Skippy wanted to make sure we knew that the bidding was still open to us. Oh goody! He's including us in the very party that we started. Anyhoo, as with The Castle, we need to write up an escalator clause bid. That is, "We will beat any offer by one thousand dollars, up to our maximum offer of . . .."

Oh, and by the way, Skippy needs the fax from us in 47 minutes.

I resent that, chop chop, we have to fax something, pronto pronto, to a grown man named Skippy, a grown man who took 37 hours to acknowledge our offer in the first place. I fuss and fume and spit and hiss and Prince keeps calm throughout, sitting quietly massaging the number pads on his 1987 calculator.

We send in our fax. The bidding will end in twelve hours.

I'm thrilled to see there is an Outback Steakhouse in town. Hoorah! Those nice folks have a gluten-free menu—including a yummy dessert, Chocolate Thunder From Down Under.

Pudge Monkey gets pretty shrill whenever I'm planning on the Chocolate Thunder indulgence. On the car ride over, Pudge whipped out the calorie counting software and ran the numbers by me: 1220 calories, 130 grams of carbohydrates, 78 grams of fat. The equivalent of one day's caloric intake. The same amount of carbs as five donuts. Five!

Who eats five donuts? She asks.

Put this way: It is the same as eating 10 pitas stuffed with 10 tablespoons of peanut butter.

She does sort of have some valid points.

I'm surprised to see Morality Monkey run to my defense. He explains that it is important to reward good behavior. We need to vote with our checkbook, we need to reward Outback for being nice enough to craft a gluten-free chocolate dessert.

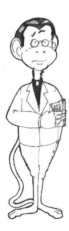

If we don't buy the dessert, then, in theory, future generations of celiacs may not enjoy this treat. Think of it, Morality said, as a living interactive culinary museum that we must preserve.

7 APRIL

P rince and I decide to skip alarm clocks and sleep until we wake up. We need to get about 500 miles out of the way today, no sense in some kind of rushed pre-sunrise scramble.

We do get the official word that The Fishbowl has been sold at a higher price to some other person. Which is fine, I guess. It sold for $204 per square foot. The people selling the house had paid $165 per square foot one year earlier. There isn't any rationality to a market like this and Prince and I are too fiscally conservative to run around and start paying New York City prices for Seattle living. You know?

We are on latte fumes. Two Starbucks stops today.

Pudge Monkey reminds me of all the times my weight has been an impediment. The guy who broke up with me because he envisioned marrying "a great pair of legs." The playwright who adored my comedic timing but said he couldn't cast me in the leading role because "audiences react better to thin, idealized beauty." The broadcast journalism school that rejected me, too tubby for TV.

Maybe that was the seed of origin for Teletubbies. It is like a weird Stanley Kubrick tragicomedy. Once you've been deemed too plump for primetime, the network keeps you on payroll and extends your health benefits and dental plan provided you don the primary colored Teletubby suit to do penance. Better still: the Teletubby suit is Hollywood's magic thin-making machine. That's probably how Jennifer Aniston and Courtney Cox got super-skinny between the second and third season of Friends.

Anyway, I tell Pudge she's dredging up things from decades ago. Things are different now, besides which, I'm no longer waddling around weighing 250 pounds. I've lost that weight and I'm a normal person now. Just slightly puffier than I'd like to be.

Pudge reminds me that there are fresh incidents. I tell her it was that once. She tells me once should be enough. I wince.

Pudge pulls up footage from the not-so-distant past. My dream job of television news anchor. The producer used to say into my earpiece, "Is it me, or did you gain about 20 pounds over the weekend, Hon? And you are on in 5... 4... 3... 2... smile! ... 1."

When my contract was up, they picked my uber-thin understudy. CNN was interested, according to my agent friend. Interested in auditioning me provided I lost 40 pounds in 6 weeks.

Pudge Monkey makes a strong case. I walk around thinking I'm not really that fat, just kind of normal and then there are lots of people on the sidelines disagreeing. Over 300 miles, I realize that this has got to be one of the dumbest things I've ever done, this yoga boot camp. Maybe this is the unity of body and mind that yoga claims. I've done the yoga, my mind now sees that I'm fat, time to turn around and go home.

In fact, if it wasn't over a thousand miles and if the Prince wasn't driving, if it was just me, I do believe I'd do a U-turn and head home.

8 APRIL

We pull into my new home-away-from-home. It took over an hour to check in, which really made me crabby. When pressed, the staff said, "We have an influx of yoga students coming in." And then I point out that I, too, am a yoga student and they looked perplexed and slightly shocked. Pudge Monkey, napping up until now, swings into action. Telling me that they are looking at my pear-shaped body and are shocked to think that I'd be some bastion of health.

Thankfully, Money Monkey is summoned for more pressing matters.

The corporate apartment people want me to sign a form that says, "Please bill my credit card for the rent every 30 days, until the dawn of time." I say, no thanks, I don't do perpetuity. (Except for Prince, but he's really handsome and he cooks dinner.)

The apartment staff person gets kind of huffy and says everyone loves, loves, loves signing that form, it is no big deal. All I want is an end date. I won't live there until the dawn of time, so why ink my name to something that says otherwise? I ask to speak to a manager. The check-in guy sighs this giant dramatic sigh and rolls his eyes as though I've asked him to crawl through broken glass to retrieve a VHS tape of Ishtar.

I'm not sure what got into me, but I snapped, "And do so with a song in your heart."

Check-in boy looks confused.

"You heard me. I'm giving you a few thousand dollars. The very least you can do is act like you want to take my money. Now. Smile."

He forces a smirk on his face and gets the manager. We iron out the kinks of the paperwork. I realized this was an expectation management issue: I expected check-in to take less time (and be less contentious) than an installment of HBO's Deadwood show.

We go to see the apartment and it is really quite spiffy and large. Two bedrooms, two bathrooms, about 1,000 square feet for just the two of us. Even a gas fireplace on a timer. I envision getting up early and supping tea before the fireplace. Meditating a little even, finding my own moment of quiet before each day of training. What a perfect idea!

We go out to the parking lot to unpack the car and from a distance, I see an Asian girl with a Nordic man—must be Yok. My new roommate.

I call out and we wave and then we hug each other and I'm weirdly very happy and excited to see her—an otherwise stranger to me. I worried she'd be a wide-eyed Holly Hobby doll, blinking and speaking like fortune cookie.

What a delightful surprise! We have lots in common, including an adult love of Hello Kitty. She's got a Master's in engineering, but is drawn to yoga inexplicably after just trying it last year, around the same time I started. She has a quick sense of humor.

Yok has managed to memorize the entire 90-minute Dialogue. This is where we differ; I'm at the halfway point. She senses my twitchy concern and says to not worry, her schooling involved nothing but rote memorization. In Thailand, that's how schools are set up. Memorize, memorize, memorize.

She's never really done any public speaking and is worried no one will understand her. I, on the other hand, have had an audience for nearly two decades and am worried that my 41-year old brain will forget what I have shoved into it. The start of a friendship, no doubt.

(Phew! Glad to check off the "friends for life" box; mission accomplished.)

SATURDAY 9 APRIL

# of days until yoga boot camp: 1

Prince and I head out to get Betty a car wash. We looked online and found one—a "car spa"—that was in the parking lot of a mall. This way we can multitask—grocery shop while Betty has spa time.

Only in California would they have spas for automobiles. Welcome to L.A., baybee. We spend most of our day sitting in traffic. We mistakenly thought six miles would be a zippy jaunt. Instead, over five hours slide away from our grasp. We do have time for a quick Costco stop and I think Prince takes comfort knowing what the new home base Costco looks like. Though, sadly, they don't have my favorite "Crunchmaster" crackers—but they do have sliced mango on sale, 2 pounds, $5.99. (Bizarrely, I cannot find my favorite prefab chai, either. Surely, I'm not looking in the right place.)

And then to the airport to drop Prince off. I cannot fathom how I'll cope without him—we were separated last summer for three weeks and I was a slobbery nose-running mess on day #16. This will be quite a challenge, though I'm hoping I'll be so very tired I simply won't have the energy for pity parties.

I get slightly lost on the way home; coming out of LAX is bizarrely complicated relative to the 1-road, then-a-left trip in. Mostly, I enjoy the drive, oogling all the swank hotels on Wilshire Boulevard. Very quickly, though, the landscape changes, and I stumble into where the Rodney King riot folks hang on Saturday nights.

White me wearing a white shirt in my white car. Good god. There was some kind of scuffle going on—it looked slightly like "West Side Story"—and the mayhem came to a standstill as the hoodlums looked up at me and Betty. Someone yelled out "Yo, whitey, maybe you should think about gettin' lost." I had to clench my jaws together to stop myself from shouting, "Oooh. Don't you have the keen eye for the patently obvious."

Felt kind of peeved as the getting lost thing screws up my yoga plan. I'm slightly wigged that I have not done yoga for over a week and I had thought I'd sneak in a class tonight so I'll be ready for tomorrow.

Instead, I didn't get home until after 10. Was so happy to run into one of my favorite comfort foods: Amy's gluten-free Mac & Cheese.

Fell asleep wrapped up in a quilt my grandma made.

SUNDAY 10 APRIL 2005

Four years ago, April 10, 2001, I was laid off, my precious precious dream television job vaporized. I had the ignominious task of calling Rosie O'Donnell to tell her that, regrettably, I would be unable to interview her the following week.

I didn't have the heart to admit it was because our machines were being repossessed and that, damn, I was lucky to find the one office phone that hadn't been disconnected. No, I just held my head high and thanked her staff for their graciousness and said we had a scheduling conflict. September 11 hadn't happened yet, so at that point, I could honestly declare April 10 to be the worst day of my life.

Four years later—I'm sitting on the floor with 200 fellow yoga teacher trainees. We sit still—as a group—for over three hours—it is a nice energy.

We are so lucky. Prior training classes were given nothing to sit on. Frankie and Laura both said a stadium chair was a "must" for my list. We walk into the massive Bikram yoga studio and there are 200 boxes laid out in four semi circles. No legs, just a T-shaped thing, but back support nonetheless. Plus which, the seat part is padded! How comfy.

We signed in, had our picture taken, got our books, assembled our chairs and listened to teachers talk about the upcoming nine weeks. Rajashree, Bikram's wife, seems to be a real-life princess. She looks like a Disney heroine, latte skin, straight long black hair down below her waist, pink flow-y Indian garb. She is also very funny. She said, "Bikram is the tiger; I am the pigeon."

Another man spoke—he's a Bikram teacher who wants to do training a second time. Not entirely altruistic—he's filming a documentary about our class. He's also looking for volunteers; he'd like to focus in on a handful of students, to closely track their experience.

TV slut that I am, I immediately preen by the camera, lengthen my neck and turn my chin to the right 15 degrees.

But, no, no, no. I don't think I shall volunteer for this gig. The documentary guy wants to focus on five students. There will be public weigh-ins and I think if I did that, Pudge Monkey would fly out of my ear canal and demand to be interviewed on the telly. No sense in giving her that kind of power.

Craig is our main guy, he's in charge of the boot camp. It seems like he's Bikram's right-hand man for the next nine weeks. Craig is a slightly stockier version of Kevin Costner (though not in the is-he-really-that-old-now? hair-thinning Upside of Anger way, more in a swaggery Field of Dreams way). Craig moved to L.A. to become a rock star and used to lift weights and, like a lot of us, was pulled to yoga in an inexplicable way. He seems really nice.

Craig gave us a few terse warnings.

Warning #1: Stay out of yoga drama. He says it is normal for a few dramatic moments to flare up, what with 200 people being pushed to their limits daily. If the drama does not directly involve you, stay away. I didn't really pay attention to the rest of what he said—I'm always on the sidelines when people get knotted up into petty fights. (Except for that one time in the college marching band, and that was just something that had to happen, it was waiting to be brought to light and I was simply the incendiary device.)

I also think, as he's smirking through this talk on "drama", that he's most likely been the center of some drama in past teacher trainings. He's as cute as Costner and in good shape and everyone's vulnerable and appears to be single. I'll bet there have been a few catfights over him.

Warning #2: Eventually, we will all be hit by what Craig calls the "yoga truck." He doesn't really explain it much more than that, just that it flattens you.

Warning #3: Bikram will do whatever he can to steal our peace. No matter what we do over the next nine weeks, do not ever allow our peace to be stolen. Remember that Bikram will do what he can to throw you off your own scent. He'll ask you in the middle of class what the next line is in the Dialogue. If he sees something screwy in your posture, he will come over to you and ask you what the hell you are doing. The end game, Craig stresses, is to not ever have your peace stolen.

Tomorrow will be 'easy'—no morning yoga class, simply start at 10 A.M. with a getting-to-know-you session with Mr. Bikram himself.

I decide that I have really got to get a handle on the Pudge Monkey chatter. Acknowledging that I have a mean monkey in my head is one thing. The next step is to just stop. I've stopped eating wheat cold turkey. I quit smoking cold turkey two summers ago. And then I dropped coffee from the regime last summer. And then milk. (But not cheese. Never, ever cheese.)

Anyhoo, the whole point is, if I can scrub those former dear-to-me items from my life, then surely, for the love of Ganesh and all other available gods, surely I can shush a monkey or two, right?

MONDAY 11 APRIL

# of days in yoga boot camp: 1

All I can say is: wheeeeeeeeee.

The first day of yoga boot camp was simply awesome.

I'll admit, I'm much more impressed with Bikram than I thought I'd be. From everything I've heard, I expected an arrogant smarty-pants. He walked into the room and there was raucous applause and he was wearing a very rockstar-ish outfit, black T-shirt and black pants and shiny Italian black shoes.

(Morality Monkey went haywire: Bikram wore shoes inside the yoga studio. Was this part of peace-stealing? Was it a trick, to see who would raise their hand and say, "Um, excuse me, Mr. YogaGuruMan, but you didn't take your shoes off?" Because, really, he probably forgot and all. So someone should help him out, right? And perhaps by not noticing, we were failing. Right?)

He taught in Tokyo for a long time. Then one night, he was summoned, put into a limo, driven to the airport, and flown to Hawaii. Richard Nixon was laid up with phlebitis and he fixed Nixon.

Bikram also insists on staying for the group getting-to-know-you thing. Which, again, surprises me. Isn't he too busy being a celebrity-fixing bendy yoga dude to sit on the floor and listen to everyone's schpiel? Doesn't Kate Hudson need another class from him?

And then I kept wondering: what's my schpiel?

There were astonishing stories. At least two addicts who got clean doing yoga. One gal had her heart rupture, just sitting there, innocent as a lamb, poof, an artery in her heart just tears. After the heart surgery, she started doing yoga. Another gal, big brown eyes and pigtails, she has fairly advanced scoliosis. When she started doing Bikram yoga six months ago, she could only put her hands on her knees in the hands-to-feet posture.

Freckly redhead from New York City, Amy. Does standup. Seems warm and nice, but also slightly shell-shocked. Almost like she was on a stage around midnight, doing her schtick and then the ceiling opened and above was a helicopter. The helicopter pilot dropped a loop around her waist, plucked her from a smoky smelly bar, and dropped her here, in yoga boot camp.

Another New Yorker—a nice warm man named Charlie. He identified himself as a former New York City firefighter. He paused and you could feel the entire group inhale for him. And then he said, "This yoga has finally allowed me to forgive." And he got quite teary and sat down and the room felt a little somber and healing-ish for a bit after that.

Well, so much for my tragicomic, "I thought my thighs were too blobby and then, speaking of lumps!, found a few in my breast and I actually don't like yoga but then it got me through the breast cancer scare, and here I am." How lame is that? Compared to drug addiction and hearts popping and rescuing charred people on September 11—what's a little cellulite, you know? I said it simply. I am a writer from Seattle.

Suddenly—it is time for our first yoga class taught by Bikram himself. I put myself in the front, my favorite place to be. Right snug up against the teaching podium. I feel pretty good about this choice. It feels like home. Plus which, since Bikram doesn't do personal corrections, there's no sense in hiding in the back row where you can't see anything.

Again, the rockstar entry. He walks in. Actually, more like he whisks into the room. He's wearing only a black Speedo and a sparkly watch. He stops by my side of the podium and puts his hair up in a topknot and then puts on a headband. This small little ritual endears him to me somehow. Most of us have some kind of pre-yoga class hair ritual—why shouldn't he?

Then the Madonna-style headset microphone comes on and he says, "Check check. One two three. Okay. Let's get started. Welcome to the Bikram torture chamber."

We slightly snicker, as a group. Suddenly, I feel awfully gassy and wonder if first row was a good choice for the first day.

In the middle of the first breathing exercise, at the very tippy top of our inhale, Bikram falls off the podium. Actually crashes on his left shoulder, almost smooshes the gal in front of the podium. Like a flash, I hear Craig's warning: Bikram will do anything to steal our peace. I refuse to fall for his bag of tricks this early, first breathing, first class, first day. I try to slyly look to my right but I don't think subtlety is a strong suit of mine.

PRANAYAMA
STANDING DEEP BREATHING

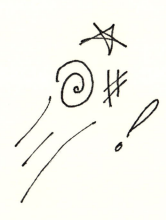

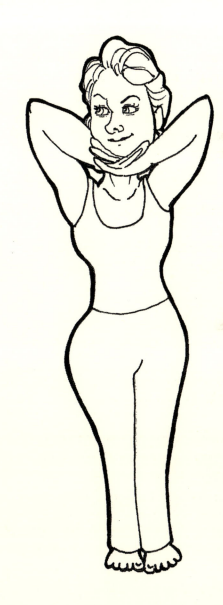

We did exhale as a group but then for about ten or seventy seconds we are all keeping our chin back on our exhale, I sense we collectively are thinking, "Nope, no peace theft from this yogi, even if I turn blue waiting for the next inhale."

The silence of our group exhale is broken by yelps and cursing; Bikram is hopping around, rubbing his elbow, face all squished up pruney in what appears to be genuine pain. I feel for him but I also still wonder if this is his usual first day schtick.

He's quite funny, and I think that everyone should laugh during class—you stretch different muscles, plus which, you can't hold your breath when you are cracking up at a joke.

So then, there I am in the first of the balancing series—Standing Head to Knee. I've never kicked out on the first set. I'm just not that type of person—that's what the bendy gumby people are for. Me, I'm happy in the first part of the posture. My standing leg seems pretty wobbly, it doesn't seem ready. I'm also a little nervous about having taken off nine days from practicing.

He booms my name into the microphone and suddenly I, a nonshy person, feel the desire to change colors, like those fish that blend with the coral when the shark is coming. I'd love to be a tawny carpet color right about now.

"Hello Miss Pink."

As per the no-peace-stealing instructions, I'm staring intently at my standing leg kneecap in the mirror. Bikram snaps his fingers in front of my face; I nearly fall straight over, mostly from the shock of my little kneecap trance being interrupted.

"Miss Pink, lock your knee. No. More. Lock your knee. Good. Now. Kick out."

I almost blurt out, "No thanks, that isn't my thing, the kicking out." Instead, I look over at him, because surely there are other Miss Pinks in the room that can actually kick out and that look like the type that kicks out.

"What da hell Miss Pink? Do you wait for everything to be perfect in your life?"

Hmm. What an excellent question. Do I wait? I think I do. I do wait. I really do—wow. A life revelation right here, right now, 30 minutes into the first class ever. He's not just a guru—he is a god!

"Misssss Piiiink. Hello. Kick out! Did you forget?"

I did forget. Am I that patently obvious—or does he read minds as well?

I have a quick flash back to my concerns about authority issues and that pledge I made to myself about never looking into his eyes.

It isn't just his eyes. It is his voice. He uses his voice very, very well. He started out singsongy, the same way you'd sing song "where are you?" when playing a game of hide-and-seek. He almost sounded sweet and a little mischievous.

Just when he's lured me into his trap, the words "kick out" sound like they are coming from a really really vengeful/bordering-on-homicidal drill sergeant.

I kick out. And I feel like a thoroughbred. I've been not-the-kicking-out-type for at least a year and it is almost as though my body has been waiting for this exact moment.

My extending leg goes exactly parallel to the floor, I'm locked out, knees snapped into place, both legs forming an upside-down 90-degree angle. Good golly! This has never happened before! Granted, I've kicked out about seven times in the past year (saving it for special occasions, I suppose)—but never like this. I feel like Cinderella, only without the shoes and the pouffy dress.

I'm in this happy zen place and I hear Bikram continue to give me instructions.

"Good. Very good Miss Pink. Now. Bend your elbows down. Down Miss Pink."

I shouldn't admit this, but: I ignored him. I knew he meant well, but I really needed to breathe and celebrate my most awesome kicking out moment. I didn't want to attempt something new and fancy and then fail and then return to feeling like a plump wanna-be. Kicking out, I felt like Homecoming Queen.

Next up, Standing Bow Pulling Pose.

Now, this posture has frustrated me in so many ways, almost like it presents to me new flavors of annoyance.

You start out balancing on one leg, then you reach around behind you and pick your right foot up in your right hand. Then you kick and supposedly your foot comes up over your head.

When I first started doing yoga, I was so anxious to blend in and look like I knew what I was doing, that I pulled on my big toe, essentially yanking my foot over my head. Then Frankie gently instructed me to think more about kicking into my hand, and then, damnit, my foot never went over my head again for about half an eternity.

Now Bikram's staring at me, and I'm thinking the first row, maybe not so much, this choice. What was I thinking? Little Miss Authority Figure Issues (years reigning: 1969-1975, 79, 80, 82, 83, 86-94) puts herself in the front row to blend? Jeesh.

(Note to self: learn better blending skills.)

He'll see that my foot doesn't go over my head and then the jig will be up. Chubby girl, row one, round like a Mentos, please take your mat and go home.

I kick like a wild mule, I don't want to go home. Oh my gosh, my toes are up over the top of my head.

"You did good Miss Pink. Now. Lock your damn knee."

The rest of class was pretty much a blur.

Also, great news. The room was not as wicked hot as I feared. It was super humid and drippy, but not nostril-hairs-on-fire hot.

I have vowed that I will not lie out. And I will never, ever leave the room.

(Well, if I'm carried out on a stretcher, that's my exception to the never-leave rule.)

But the drippiness made me feel really thirsty. I think I drank a little too much water (rank amateur mistake), so I felt pretty pukey when upside down. But, even with bile in my throat and puddles of sweat in my ears, I did not leave the room, I didn't lie down and, most importantly, I did not ack on famous Bikram.

I'm so blessed to have been trained by such a good studio. There were all kinds of moaning and puking and leaving the room and bawling. At least four crying yogis by my count. Frankie and Laura were right—the nine days off was perfect. I felt like a frisky pony, prancing on my mat, waiting for the starting bell of each posture.

We had a dinner break and then some getting-to-know-you people to finish. Bikram sat in a very comfy chair with an orange and pink towel and then women rotated brushing his hair and rubbing his now-injured elbow.

He was so pleased with our progress on our first day that he let us go home early.

Got a load of laundry done.

TUESDAY 12 APRIL

# of days in yoga boot camp: 2

Today was our first full day. Therefore, our first sense of what kind of mayhem ensues when, right after the morning class, 150 sweaty yoginis are trying to shove into the bathroom. We all need to either pee or shower or both. And the four-sink, six-stall, eight-shower bathroom just cannot accommodate so many demands from so many people. There's a line to get into the room and so I decide that I'll mingle first and get fresh air and eat some lunch and then shower once rush hour has calmed down.

I'm out in the garage with this Jason actor guy and he has listened to me say my Dialogue. Actor Jason seems very self assured and he rocks back on his heels and says, "Wow, I can't wait to take your class," and just as I'm about to flatter myself, he quips, "You'll be done with class in less than 60 minutes at that pace." He slightly had a point but I feel overly critiqued. Who made him Mr. FancyPants?

I'm heading back into the building and a gal from the front desk who looks like Audrey Hepburn, long neck and all, comes running out and says, "Bikram is looking for you."

I ask why and she says you just go when summoned. Fuck. I made this goal of avoiding the man and this is not helping. I dash into the room and Bikram is being tractioned. He has a rolled-up towel under his chin and another rolled up towel wrapped around each ankle and these big burly guys are pulling really hard and he's making oomphy tractioning sounds.

So I walk up and stand there, listening to the sounds of the showers still running, listening to the tinkly sounds of women laughing like they are all old school chums, wondering why I'm here and why don't I make friends well?

I thought again about the "you'll make friends for life" claim and I realize that there won't be any friends left for me—all the friendship is being claimed in the clubby humid bathroom and, honestly, if I were the kind of girl that chummed right up to people, I wouldn't be here right now, would I?

Bikram looks up at me, his usually dark debonair face all squished up like a naughty chipmunk. The eyes sparkle. And dance. And wink. And bedazzle.

"Who da hell are you?"

"Um."

(Which name do I give him? First name? Or last name?)

"Who?"

"Um. Okay. Sorry. Pink. Ah. Miss Pink."

"Why are you here?"

"Sorry?"

"Why are you standing here?"

"Right. See. Girl. Front desk. She said come."

I'm simply awful sometimes. Most times, I'm unflappable. But when I lose my mission, I start blurting out thought pellets like I've been possessed by a Morse code ghost.

"No. No. No. Idiot!"

See, I knew I'd hate this guy. Why am I the idiot? Admittedly I did sound a little slow-ish, but I think calling me an idiot is harsh. Bite tongue. Blend. Breathe.

Bikram warmly smiles up at me. His voice is soft, as though he's the patient father explaining, again, to his dim-witted child, how to tie shoes.

"No. Not you. I tell her to get the girl who look like you. She helped my elbow. So please. Go get the girl who look like you but isn't you."

There's probably some Indian fairy tale that starts out just like this.

There I am, she who doesn't always make friends, going around, asking, "Hi. Who looks like me but isn't me?"

Amy from New York found the humor in my predicament. Threw her head back and laughed. I asked her if she had done improvisational comedy—turns out we had some friends in common. Isn't that amazing, that six degrees of separation thing?

Surprisingly, as the bathroom emptied, I got my answer. A gal named Holly with white blonde hair and big blue eyes—she's a massage therapist and the gal who fixed Bikram's elbow. I was tired and annoyed and all I could blurt out was, "You look nothing like me at all!"

Now for an embarrassing confession. Probably shouldn't even write this down. I'm such a bozo some times.

So I was out practicing Dialogue and then ran around asking everyone to find the girl the king wanted—and then—I heard silence. I went into the bathroom and it was empty!

Hoorah—my plan, although slightly thwarted—would now unfold. I got out my shower gel and leave-in five-minute deep conditioner and the water was hot and I was loving my sometimes-hermitic life. No swarms of women, no mounds of towels, no line, no waiting, just me and eight showers.

I think to myself, solitariness has its upside. See? I get a quiet shower and they are all eating lunch now.

Sure is quiet though.

I cannot believe I'm such a genius! I mean, seriously, I don't think I'm necessarily the brightest bulb on the Christmas tree, but it seems hard to imagine that out of 150 gal classmates, only I had this ingenious idea.

Maybe I am that smart?

Nah.

Probably just from nearly two decades living in New York, I've learned how to survive.

Got my deep conditioner on, massaging my scalp, falling in love with my very own savvy. Then. Awful sound. The microphone in the big hot room is being turned on. I hear "testing," followed by tap tap tap.

No reason to panic. People are probably going to practice using a microphone before we start reciting Dialogue.

And then I hear Craig say, "Thank you all for being on time. If you are ever late, it will be counted as an absence. And absences very much impact your ability to graduate."

Oh fuck oh fuck oh fuck, I'm not the brightest bulb! I'm the bulb that fell out onto the floor, the bulb that gets eaten by the dog. What to do? Stay in here the rest of the day? I mean, if I go in there, they will all know I'm late. Oh god.

My new compadres will see me saunter in and they'll think, "Oh, she was probably the girl that smoked pot and missed frog dissection in high school."

I quickly rinse the remaining four minutes of conditioner out of my hair. Damnit. It was a five-pack treatment and will only work properly with each packet soaking in for five full minutes.

Right as I'm shoving everything back into my gym bag, I hear some scuffled running down the hallway and there's this girl with a jaunty hat on and another really blonde girl with glasses and they squeal into the room and Craig says, "Hello ladies. Care to join us today?"

Oh god. He is going to be one of those ball-busting types.

He shines the bare light bulb on these two girls. They totally look like the kind that sat in the back of the bus and had flasks and played cards on the way to school. You know, the fun ones.

All 200 students are sitting in those comfy purple back-supporting chairs (can't wait to e-mail Frankie and tell her we got it good here)—so late entries are just patently obvious.

I wait for Craig's skewering of these two gals to die down. Maybe he's like a Duraflame log. The temper just burns for exactly four minutes and then, poof, there's just nothing left.

Craig returns to his schpiel and I slink in unnoticed. I slide down the back wall. My hair is dripping wet and, quite frankly, I smell fabulous. No two ways around it: I ooze clean, I emit beams of soapy shower fun.

Craig hands the microphone over to someone else and walks back to me and I'm looking into his eyes and I'm mentally pleading, oh, dude, please oh please know that I'm not a flask back-bus gal, I'm not, I'm just . . . you know . . . I . . ..

He walks straight up to me and leans in and I squint my eyes, the way my kitten Gigi squints to prepare for a bad-kitty spritz from the spray bottle.

Craig leans in even closer and whispers, "Don't be late again. No sitting against the wall please. Move up into one of the backjacks. You must be involved; this is your community."

With that, he turned and walked away and I exhaled for about two minutes.

Now for Bikram's blessing of each teacher trainee.

All 200 of us are sitting in 4 semicircle arcs. Bikram is in the front, in his special chair with Craig on his right side and that gal that looks like Audrey Hepburn on his left. From time to time, Audrey alternates between brushing his hair and rubbing his elbow.

Three students stand facing the audience; they are the mock class. One by one, each student goes up, takes the mike, and delivers the Dialogue.

I was going to stay in the back row and just get the feel of how this is all going to go. Then I remembered: Frankie recommended that when it was time to perform the memorized Dialogue bits, to just get up and go at the beginning. She said she often waited until the end to go up and deliver the Dialogue and wished she had just gotten it out of the way.

The first dozen students that went were really very strong and I briefly considered the very real possibility that, for the first time in my life, I may have oversold myself on my skills. Nonetheless, I throw myself into the line of people waiting to go up and deliver the Dialogue.

Bikram minces no words. One gal said the Dialogue waaaay too slow and Bikram said "Not bad. Only, I pay 10 dollars for your class because it is 3 hours long and I have to quit my job to take your 3-hour class and I cannot afford a 20 dollar class any more."

I do feel uncharacteristically nervous, especially given Bikram's blunt feedback. I'm reminding myself of all the times I was horrendously so less prepared than I am right now. Those times all turned out just fine.

Like the first job interview in New York. The guy was quite flippant and snarky and barked out, "Why the hell should I hire some broad from way down below the damn Mason-Dixon line?" and all I could do was bite back with, "Why the hell wouldn't you?"

And the first time I had to give a trading recommendation to a room full of 300 sweaty men.

Or the first time I marched in the band with a saxophone instead of my beloved piccolo. All those times—I was too stubborn to say, "Nope, I just can't do this." I took a giant breath and faked it.

My turn. The microphone is handed to me and all of the sudden, I'm right back to the Sweatbox, the first time I said the Dialogue in front of Frankie. Shaking like a Vermont maple leaf in the middle of a gusty October day. My kneecaps become Play Doh. The microphone weighs about 60 pounds.

I breathe and thinking of my near-miss with Craig, I stare into Bikram's eyes, as if to say "Okay, pal, I don't frighten easily." His eyes are intense. The sparkle of an opal and yet black like a black diamond but melted into liquid. My heart redoubles its efforts to relocate into the base of my throat.

I think my knees actually knock and I'm relieved that I'm wearing long pants and you can't see my wibbly joints.

I tell myself, just one sentence at a time and breathe. Pudge Monkey startles me; she reminds me to turn sideways by 30 degrees so I'll at least look thin to Bikram. Money Monkey shoves Pudge out of the way—he reminds me that, next to my car, this is the largest investment of my life. Poor performance here could signify a long-term trend of low rate of return on said investment.

Three sentences into it, I catch a glimpse of the garage guy, Jason, out of the corner of my eye. He was right. I was too fast in the garage and I'm not sure, but I think Jason was sending me a "slow down, you are fine" message.

I took another breath and slowed the tempo down about 25 percent. No bloopers, no errors, just every single word of Dialogue came out of my mouth. Even the part about "flower petal blooming."

Bikram looked astonished when I finished. He paused for a while, for what felt like 17 hours, and then he said, "I have no negative comments."

Another giant ball of space without any sound.

Crap. "No negative comments" isn't exactly a ringing endorsement.

I look over at Jason again. Breathe, his eyes say, don't forget to breathe.

Bikram swallows a couple of times and then continues.

"Everything is perfect. Timing is perfect. If you know all the Dialogue, you teach class tonight instead of me. Yes?"

I declined demurely. Secretly, though, kicked myself for not having memorized the whole Dialogue. Damnit. If only I could borrow Yok's brain for just one evening.

Bikram asked me a lot of questions. How long did I study? How long have I done his yoga? Which studio sent me?

Chest puffed with pride, I said the Sweatbox in Seattle.

He nodded slowly, as if it all made sense now, and said, "Seattle very good."

Hoorah!

For class that evening, I was at "my spot" again today. So was Emily. She's a ballet dancer from New York City. Looks like she just got off paw's turnip truck from the farm. Freckles, red hair, creamy flawless skin, big warm open honest smile. She's right behind me in the second row.

Bikram taught the evening class. He gave me so many corrections. I'm not sure if I should feel honored to get his individual attention—or worried that he's thinking about tossing me out on my ear.

In Awkward Pose, I had always thought that if your ankles were wobbly, to just stay in that spot and not sit down more.

"Miss Piiiiink. You have to sit your hips down. All the way down. More down. Heels up now. Hips down, Miss Pink. Did I say hips up? No. I tell you heels up."

He takes the time to spell the word, haitch ee ee ell.

And then in Standing Bow, "Miss Pink. You do good. Now kick harder. And reach with your fingers like this, look at me, like this, juuuum." And he demonstrates his shoulder going out of the socket.

I attempt the juuuum shoulder thing, and look over to see if that's right.

He bellows out, "What are you doing Miss Pink? Don't look at me. Reach and look in the mirror, Miss Pink."

WEDNESDAY 13 APRIL

# of days in yoga boot camp: 3

Bikram's wife Rajashree taught the morning class. Such a delight. She seems to float, somehow. And while Bikram's voice has the rasp of Danny DeVito, Rajashree's voice sounds like—like, okay, you are on your deathbed and then you float towards the white light and you are scared and there's a willowy angel that greets you at the end of the light tunnel and she holds out her warm hand and says, "there, there, don't be frightened." She sounds like that.

Lots more weeping in class, so much so that I almost feel left out. Maybe I should just try really hard to cry to get it over with? I try to think of sad things. Like that precious silver mouse ring my Aunt Shirley sent as a birthday gift. Promptly lost it and cried for at least a week.

Nothing.

Having to euthanize Dante the kitty in his sixth month due to some awful kitty cancer.

Nada.

Having to break up with best-sex-ever boyfriend, who shrugged and said "Shush, shush, sweetie. Don't cry. Dante was just a dumb cat."

Zip.

My best-friend-for-life Annie Stevens dying way too young, at age 25.

Zilch.

Running through the names of all my friends who died in the World Trade Center: Andy. Bill. Brendan. Cruikshank. Dean. Ira.

Slight bit of a lip tremor but zero tears.

I go darker: did they jump? Or did they stay behind and suffocate? Do the surviving spouses know that answer? Do they tell their children?

Three little tears squeak out. Perhaps the year of crying jags simply depleted my tear pool.

Mum's birthday today. Was feeling kind of sad about the possibility of not being able to at least call her. Bikram gave us an unexpected break in the afternoon. He walked by and saw me and stopped. He stooped down and put my face in his hands. He asked, "Miss Pink, why so sad?"

I was sad it was my mum's birthday and I wasn't sure I'd be able to call.

"What's her name?"

Why would he care? Isn't that odd? I think so.

"Um. Ruth."

"Please go call your mother and tell Ruth I wish her a happy birthday as well."

Quite nice, really, for a fancy yoga man, no?

Long long day of posture clinic—which goes like this. Four volunteers stand up in front of Bikram, a mock "class" of students. One teacher-in-training gets up and delivers about 60 seconds of memorized Dialogue and the students do as instructed. Mostly boring. But, sometimes comical when things get mixed up. Today, one guy said "push your right hip all the way out until your hip goes through your rib cage."

Bikram taught the evening class. Starts staring at me funny during Eagle. Says, "Miss Pink, interlock your damn fingers and then go back and forth."

I really have no idea what he's talking about. My fingers aren't anywhere close to each other so interlocking seems physically impossible. I move my fingers a little, to indicate that I've heard his instructions. I'd so love to ask him some questions, but, no sense in breaking some protocol on day number three of boot camp.

We go to the other side of Eagle. He snaps his fingers in front of my face.

"Hello, do you hear me Miss Pink? Look, go like this."

And he shows me how to do it; it makes sense.

I look at my two hand pressed together. My left hand is nice and straight. My right hand fingers are by my wrist.

GARURASANA
EAGLE

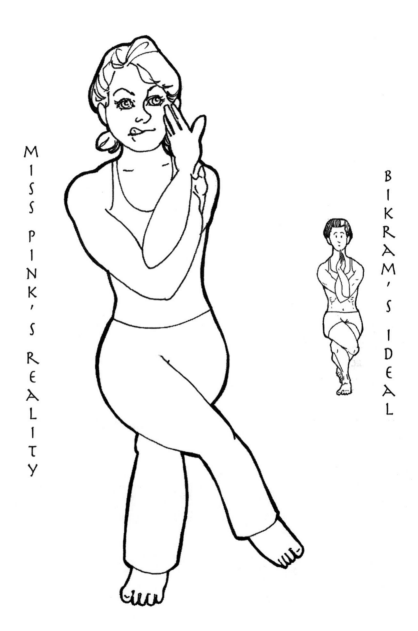

MISS PINK'S REALITY

BIKRAM'S IDEAL

Sigh.

I peek over at Matmate Emily; her hands are perfectly pressed together as though she is clapping.

"Like this Miss Pink, pulllll your right fingers up with your left fingers."

I quirk my eyebrow up at him, thinking loudly "Really now?"

I do his bidding and oh my gosh, my left fingers really did pull up my right wrist-tickling fingers. Wow. Didn't see that coming at all.

"Now, move them back and forth. Usually 10 times is what you tell your students, but Miss Pink, you need more time, move them back and forth 15 times."

I shoot him an "I don't get that at all" look and then he shows me again. It is a weird little wrist motion, wrists are flopping back and forth.

I do the back and forth thing three times. My back shoulder blade wings are burning from the back-and-forth action.

Phew. To my immediate relief, Bikram's head turns to the other side of the room. I cease backing-and-forthing, mostly because I've sort of lost count and I don't want to miss what comes next.

Without ever looking my way, he says, "Miss Pink, you only did it three times. You owe me 12 times on the second set."

Good golly, the man has eyes like a fly. Those multi-faceted orbs that catch images from all around.

After class, lots more posture clinic. Each and every teacher-trainee must get Bikram's blessing. With 200 people traipsing through, we stayed until way past midnight. Didn't get home until after one in the morning.

THURSDAY 14 APRIL

# of days in yoga boot camp: 4

For trying to avoid the man, I'm doing an awful job.

During the lunch break, Bikram came up to me, rubbing his elbow—the one he injured falling off the podium.

He held out his wounded wing to me and those liquid black diamond eyes seem very round-shaped and he looked quite pitiable.

He said, "Ooh, Miss Pink, my elbow hurts bad." The arm is dangling between us.

Hmm.

Am I supposed to touch it? Should I kneel first?

I mean, seriously, what is guru etiquette? Maybe you shouldn't ever touch your guru—I think I read that in National Geographic once. Or was it National Enquirer? Definitely National Somethingorother magazine. Or journal. One of them. Bad luck, I think.

If I were in a supermarket trying to buy avocados and a glistening-in-sweat 60-year-old man, dressed in nothing but a Speedo, approached me and asked me to rub his arm, I'd think him a pervert and alert security.

(I'd probably also leave the store in a huff, unless the avocados were a good deal, then I'd have to rethink the exit strategy.)

Then again, I'm thinking I can't just decline.

How would that sound: "You know, Mr. Bikram, see, I'd rather not."

I burble out something about how I'm sorry it still hurts. The elbow dangles awkwardly now, we are frozen in this bizarre tableau in the center hallway 10 minutes before class starts.

Then I remember Bikram's oft-cited quote: "It's never too late, it's never too bad, you're never too old, you're never too sick to start from scratch once again. "

I say, tentatively, "You know, it is never too late, never too bad . . .."

His eyes narrow and he makes some kind of pshaw noise and says he has no time.

"But wouldn't Eagle help with elbow issues?"

Now I feel silly. Who the hell do I think I am? Me, round writer chick, telling the king of yogis what to do. Oh god, if only the earth would swallow me right now.

My sentence and his elbow are now both midair danglers, competing for space.

"Come take class with us tonight!" I blurt out with way too much enthusiasm.

"No. I have no time. I have so much to do."

"You are the boss. You should make time."

"No, no, no."

He seems quite adamant and his dangly arm returns to his side. He rubs it hard and winces.

"But your yoga fixes everything, right? You know, everyone is so tired and it would be exciting to have you come and take the class with us."

He says something and I don't really hear it because I'm just so appalled at myself. While I'm at it, why don't I call Alan Greenspan up and tell him to consider subscribing to the Wall Street Journal? Or call Emeril and tell him that a little garlic goes a long way. What is wrong with me?

I'm in my spot for the evening class and the Audrey Hepburn girl from the front desk (and the same gal who brushed Bikram's hair last night) —she came up and asked if I would move my mat.

Class is about to start and I'm thinking, well, fuck, so now Audrey Hepburn is going to get the good spot and I'll get shoved under the heater and I'll be screwed and yet Audrey has an air of import and so I say kind of lamely, "But where will I go?"

She laughs and says, "I just need you to move to your left about a foot. Bick is going to take class and you are in front of his spot."

Bick. Who the hell is this Bick person?

Then I see the pink and orange "Hot Stuff" towel and my heart valves flutter simultaneously.

That Bick.

The confusion is on the pronunciation of his name. Some people say Bick-rawm and others (myself included) pronounce it Beek-rum and, good god, I'm probably not even saying his name right.

I had to keep reminding myself that Craig told us Bikram would try to steal our peace. Much easier to ignore him amidst 200 students, sitting in the next-to-last row. Much harder to ignore him when he's six inches from the back of your yoga mat. And impossible when he says things like, "Hey. Psst. Miss Pink. What da hell is dat? Didn't I tell you to sit alllll the way down?"

He did the postures and came out early and said things like, "Damn, I forgot how hard I make this series." He reminded me a little of Danny DeVito with a zing of Robin Williams zaniness.

He started walking around, trying to make people fall over. Towards the end, in floor bow, he picked people up by the toes and then their bodies went from awkward U-shapes to beautiful teardrops.

Matmate Emily got picked up and spun around in Full Locust and she looked like a kid loving her first teacup spin at the amusement park. I think if I were thinner, I would definitely have raised my hand to volunteer for that.

FRIDAY 15 APRIL

# of days in yoga boot camp: 5

Really interesting day.

The morning class was taught by a woman named Cindy. She has been doing yoga since the mid-1970s with Bikram. We had been forewarned that her classes were brutal. It was a bit hotter than usual and longer than usual, but a lot of fun.

Noon lecture was a special guest, Dr. Lilly. Bikram sang her praises all week. He credits her for saving his voice. Twenty years ago, Bikram was told he'd have to stop teaching in order to save his voice, after he developed some sort of growth on his vocal chords. Dr. Lilly came to Bikram's rescue. She specializes in speech therapy, so all day long we were pretty anxious for her hands-on voice training.

Dr. Lilly started the workshop with each teacher trainee grabbing the mike and saying a few words about themselves, just a random thought or two, so she could get a sense of their speech and body language.

One skinny pigtailed gal named Sarah introduced herself and made a crack about Awkward Pose. I'm pretty sure she's the girl with the wicked scoliosis. She said, "As much as I love the series, oh, my gosh, what's with Awkward? That posture can just destroy you."

Dr. Lilly seemed offended and gave Sarah a lecture about the importance of always saying nice things about your party hosts and how it is rude to criticize Bikram's yoga. We are in his home and so this is no place to ever say anything bad.

Pigtail Sarah looked like she was going to cry.

A few more students go up and say things and Dr. Lilly seems to hit the nail on the head in terms of how they are speaking.

Then, that girl with the hat who was late when I was showering - her name is Jaimie. It is her turn to go up to the microphone and she has her jaunty hat on and she is standing kind of like a slouchy petulant just-been-grounded teenager. Jaimie starts to speak but Dr. Lilly interrupts her immediately to correct her posture. (Now, see, if it were me, I'd have to straighten the hat first!)

Jaimie took offense at the posture correction and then she got defensive. There's this sticky to-fro between the two women and it feels like it will never end. Suddenly, the needle jerks off the vinyl record as Jaimie snarks out, "Listen sweetheart, you don't know everything."

Ooopsie.

In BikramLand, even after a week, his habit of calling boys "boss" and girls "sweetheart" has rubbed off. Yet all of the sudden, in this context, it sounds horrifically wrong.

Speaking of wrong, I'm looking at Jaimie's hat and it appears to be wool or a wool blend. Isn't it hot?

Dr. Lilly corrected her and said sweetheart was derogative. Jaimie said no, Bikram calls everyone that. The room seemed to be filling with the word sweetheart and the tension was reaching all the way up to the end of the keyboard, shrill and demanding.

Somehow they manage to disengage and Jaimie sat down and no one really exhaled.

A few minutes later, a guy named J. Michael had his turn at the microphone. He said that sarcasm and irony were in fact the hidden truths of existence and, therefore, the straightest path to self-awareness and acceptance. I was still wondering about how that worked, was he right, was the eternal "Why am I here?" question answered that simply? And as I'm spinning through my thought processor, Dr. Lilly had both J. Michael and JauntyHatJaimie ejected from the room. So I think I missed something.

Dr. Lilly went into a long segue about expectations and relatives surviving World War II, and then there was a smattering of tentative applause and then she did a book signing and she left.

Apparently, though, she left quite angry. She told Bikram that she will never come back to help out and I do wonder if she got a speaker's fee and if so, does it get refunded? Or, is it that Bikram now needs to pay her extra hazard pay?

I was talking with Pigtail Sarah and Leo (this very sweet burly man who stands outside the front door every day like a bouncer at a club)—and Bikram was walking through the room, asking what happened. No one really answered his question. And, to be honest, while I was still wondering why you'd wear a wool cap in a hot room, I was still deep in thought about J. Michael's statement regarding sarcasm and truth and inner zenniness.

Bikram's getting nothing but deer-in-headlights blank stares. He sees me and snaps his fingers and says, "You. Miss Pink."

(Instinctively, I lock my knees.)

"You will tell me the truth."

I'm not certain why I end up in these spots in life—the Mrs. Kravitz/hall monitor—but here I am again.

I told Bikram that I think things got misinterpreted and that the one girl did kind of come across as flippant. However, to be fair to everyone, I said I thought Dr. Lilly got too upset and then the guy said sarcasm led to peace. Bikram said he had not been able to figure out who the girl was. I said she was the girl with the hat.

"She wears a hat?"

Yes.

"A hat on her head?"

Yes.

"Why? Is she cold?"

See-it isn't just me. Hats and hot yoga don't mix.

Maybe she's balding and embarrassed. Nah. Can't be, she's too young for that.

Bikram snaps his fingers and says, "Bring her to me."

I go into the big room and I find JauntyHatJaimie and I tell her Bikram wants to see her, and she says she's in the middle of a conversation and can't I see that I just walked into the middle of it. Hmm. She had a point. But I think he's got a quick temper and he did ask me to do this one thing—and, quite frankly, after a week of mishaps with this man, I'd like to put a cherry on the week and then fade into obscurity.

I asked her to come with me and she looked pretty annoyed and I said meekly, look, he asked, and I'm here and let's just get this over with and I'm walking down the hall with her and I'm just dying to know all about the hat. First off, there are many hats, and I'd like to know how many hats there are. Secondly, she matches each hat with each outfit quite fetchingly and how does she do that? And, thirdly, she's from Montreal—how does she travel and put hats into a suitcase and not have them get smooshy?

And, lastly, how old is she? She could be early 20s. That's the only explanation I can find for someone doing yoga all the livelong day, laundry at night and still be stylish and plucky in between.

Morality Monkey is reminding me that blurting things out usually gets me into trouble, like the time I met that CNBC anchor and said, "My! You are so much shorter in person. That's sad, really. You even sound tall on the television."

Instead I go with the standard, "So, how old are you?" And she says 30 and I'm just shocked. Her skin doesn't say 30 at all, so then I have a long list of skin care questions to add to the fashion questions and, really, at 30, shouldn't you just be a little more ready to kind of suck it up and not be lippy to a guest speaker?

I blurt out, "Thirty? Wow. No kidding. You might be screwed. Nice hat though."

I smile wincingly at her, partially out of pity for her situation but mostly out of pity for my poor mouth and its ability to just shoot things out randomly.

Morality Monkey happily replays the tape in my head. There I am, saying, "You are screwed. Nice hat." Good god.

Our evening class was taught by a young pup named Josh.

Before Josh started class, Bikram came in and gave us a long and somber talk, reminding us to leave our egos at the door. He told us again and again that he was simply too sad to be angry about the Dr. Lilly event.

Right in the middle of a serious and determined balancing series, the back door swings wide open. In blows a fresh burst of cool air – and Bikram. He's literally bouncing with glee. The Chinese version of his Bikram book has just been published.

Even from half a football field away, you can see there's a glint in his eye. Like a cartoon character that gets a little star accompanied by a "ting" sound. That kind of glint.

Treated myself to a most excellent sushi fest and, more importantly, another load of laundry out of the way.

Saturday 16 April

# of days in yoga boot camp: 6

We've survived Rajashree and Emmy and Bikram and Cindy. All that's left is Craig.

Reputedly one of the toughest teachers around. And allegedly obsessed with aforementioned thigh-busting Awkward Pose.

And . . . we face him at 7:30 in the morning on Saturdays. Uck.

We are all tired and squinty eyed. Except for that guy Leo the bouncer. He reminds me a little of Bruce Willis. The older, balder Bruce, not the young Moonlighting Bruce.

Leo is also probably twice as tall as Bruce.

I once saw Bruce Willis. He was filming in New York and they had closed 8th Street and I was meeting the Prior Husband at the BBQ place on 8th and the movie dude was all rent-a-cop on me and telling me I can't cross. The movie people are trying to figure out how to "recreate" New York traffic. Thanks to their movie idiocy, Broadway is at an utter standstill for almost two miles, all the way up through Times Square.

It isn't like I want to walk through a precious Die Hard scene, it's just that this is pre-cell phone and I pay taxes out the yingyang and the very least I can do is walk down the street about 600 feet. So the movie dude says, okay, fine, but don't cross to the south side of the street. See? That's where Bruce is. Where? I'm squinting. There. Really? In the distance I see this short balding guy in jeans and a t-shirt and he looks like he's wearing those earthy Birkenstock shoes. And then I said, "Gosh, he's short. I thought he was tall, like six feet or something. He isn't as short as that shrimp on CNBC. But, dang, he's one little fella."

Basically, Leo has the same facial structure and twinkly eyes as Bruce. He's simply as tall as Bruce Willis should be.

Leo looks like a bouncer. He's always smiling and happy, standing on the right-hand side of the entrance to the yoga college. He's quite muscle-y and, honestly, almost every day I see him, I'm astonished that he's doing yoga. If he were less smiley and shaved less often, he'd be great in a police line up. Line up yes, yoga class—not on your life.

Craig started class by stating his rules. We are to only drink water when instructed to do so. We will not leave the room. If we leave the room, it will be marked as an absence. Absences, he reminds us, will be a large obstacle to leaving here with a diploma.

The water thing really freaked me out. The second he made that kingly proclamation, a little cotton field grew inside my mouth. Parched. So dry, I couldn't even swallow.

I worked harder in postures for that very reason. For the first time ever, I attempted to bring my forehead to my knee in Standing Head to Knee. I realized that if I got my head all the way down, I could lick my leg, which was quite sweaty. King Craig said nothing about licking of one's sweat.

DANDAYAMANA JANUSHIRASANA
STANDING HEAD TO KNEE

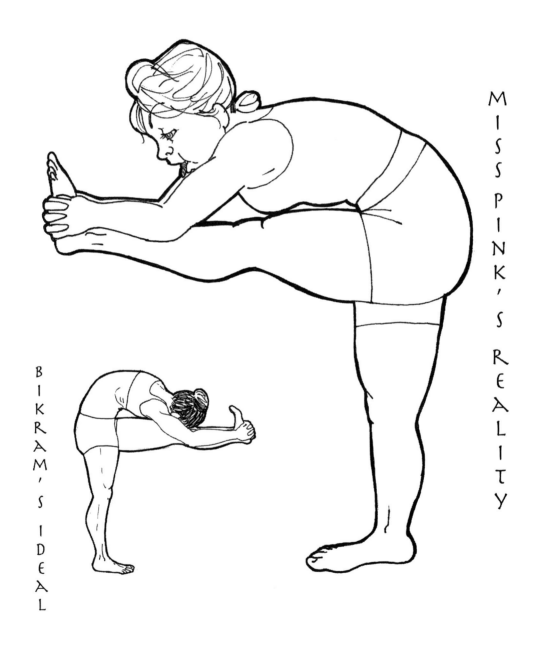

MISS PINK'S REALITY

BIKRAM'S IDEAL

Funny, all week there've been people fainting and laying out on the sofa in the lobby and crying and everything and I've half wondered if I was doing the yoga wrong. Been feeling really fine and rock solid, actually.

Ha. Came home from Craig's class and was immediately ill. Food leaving me oh-so-quickly, I'm shaky and sweaty and can barely stand and I'm desperate to call and cancel my chiropractor appointment. I drive quickly, not sure my colon will hold out for the two-mile ride.

I don't usually like discussing bodily fluids, but I also could hear my colon sending out distress flares and I felt it best to be up front with my new chiropractor. He nodded and said it was good that I was getting rid of toxins. He said he had a way to help bring it full circle. He put me in these giant pants—that were made like a blood pressure cuff. He zipped me in and then turned the pants on and they puffed up like a blood pressure machine—and I fell asleep. Woke up feeling much better and the tummy had stopped yowling.

Went to Blockbuster—rented movies—and stayed in bed the rest of the day. Eyes felt heavy around three or so, and next thing, it was nine at night. Quick dinner, called Prince and then fell back into a deep dead zone and slept another 14 hours.

MONDAY 18 APRIL

# of days in yoga boot camp: 8

Back up to the microphone to recite more Dialogue. This time we were doing the second half of Half Moon—only in front of Craig instead of in front of Bikram.

Apparently I did quite well. Craig took off his headset microphone, bowed, and handed the mike to me. Lots of applause. When the applause stopped, he put the mike back on and said, "Please make us mere mortals feel better and tell me you have had some kind of professional training."

I reluctantly confessed to radio and TV experience. As much as television was my dream job, the one thing I've found over the years is that there's this odd dance you do with nonTV people.

When you first say you work in television, people ooh and aaah and gush and get pink in the cheeks, as though they are flustered. Then they ask, "Have I seen you in something?"

When I've puffed my chest and crowed, "Yes. Surely you caught me on Fox this morning"—then there's the niggling of details, which show, what time, and slowly the pink drains out of their cheeks and then they become disappointed. Oh, okay, not a real television star, just some dweeb on at six in the morning.

The second choice is to be demure, wave my hand, make a pshaw noise, and insist that it isn't anything big, just a little hobby. An odd attempt to deflect envy, if you will. As if to say, "No, no, really, I'm barely on at all and, honestly, who is up that early in the morning anyway?" The problem with this approach is that the cheeks pinken even more as the nonTV human is now convinced fame is right in their palm, they can touch it and almost smell it and they want the details, damnit.

The whole 'what do you do for a living?' thing became so fraught that I eventually told people, "I'm an editor"—just to avoid the whole TV dance.

But I realize that scads of celebrities have put their sweat on this exact floor, so there's no reason in hiding anything. I said I was a financial journalist in radio and TV and Craig nodded. He wanted to know what that meant—what did I say when I went on air? I said it was sort of like the Vanna White of the Nasdaq, and that seemed to have struck a chord.

He asked for a demo of what I used to say. Almost as reflexive as sneezing, I recited my little schpiel on how the closing price of gold in Hong Kong affects the opening price of gold in Chicago. Again, thunderous applause.

I feel like crying big, plinky, happy tears. I don't get a single bad vibe from the room and I smile to myself as I return to my comfy purple back jack.

Funny how life works out, isn't it? All those years I banged my forehead bloody against the broadcast wall, desperate for a promotion, desperate for recognition of all I had to offer. Yet all I got was years of being told I was too chubby, my hair too fuzzy, my skin too blotchy and unpredictable, someone of my girth couldn't possibly be worthy of reading the TelePrompTer verbatim.

And now, here I am, performing word-by-word recitings in front of 200 yogis, and the only one whining about my looks is me and Pudge Monkey. So I think I've hit my stride.

Out in the garage for lunch. The garage has a nice counter-culture feel to it. About 90 percent of the students opted to stay in the dorm-style housing provided by Bikram and then use Bikram-provided vans to shuttle back and forth.

Those of us that opted for something a little different are driving our own cars and staying in housing we selected. I think the main difference is our socializing options. The dorm people are living in clumps of 5 and van-ing in clumps of 10—so there are lots of ways they are being forced to interact with people.

Us garage folks though, not so much.

I do like it in the garage, though. It is dark and cool—a welcome balm after leaving the big hot room. Plus which, there's a hidden bathroom that's always empty—and a microwave.

There's a tall gal standing back in the corner, eating a giant ruby red strawberry and struggling mightily to spit out the Dialogue. Her name is Julie, she's from Canada and she likes to golf.

She congratulates me on my success of the day and asks if I have any tips for her. I'm embarrassed to admit all the crazy things I tried—writing the Dialogue out by hand, listening to it on my iPod, typing it over and over. I tell her she's building a muscle memory of reciting it clutching the Dialogue book and when I go to look at her book, her knuckles tighten and her eyes get big and she pleads, "No, no, no, I neeeed it."

Hmmm.

Feeling prank-ish, I take the book from her and tell her she can't have it back until she recites five sentences in a row. She sputters a bit but eventually three and a half sentences sneak out, despite Julie's best efforts to the contrary.

She says she's thankful for my help and then when we are walking back to the college, I wonder—maybe this is why I'm not making friends? I probably shouldn't have taken her book and maybe that's a mean nonfriendly thing to do and she waves at me as she goes over to the corner where two other gals have saved her a seat.

TUESDAY 19 APRIL

# of days in yoga boot camp: 9

Emmy taught this morning's class. She's the self-described "older than god" woman who has been with Bikram since his arrival in the U.S. in the 1970s. She's very sweet and likes to tell long stories while you are holding a posture. So it is a weird experience of incredible envelope-pushing with a sweet grandma voice chattering away gently.

Incredibly fatigued. After the 9:30 A.M. class, we break for an hour, then head into anatomy class. The classes are held in the same room where we do the hot yoga—so the room is still sort of hot and muggy. Then they turn the lights out to show slides—and heads start nodding.

Somehow, I did stay awake through the anatomy lecture. After anatomy was Emmy's lecture on pain. People rave about it. Even Laura (or was it Frankie?) said the pain lecture was nothing short of spectacular.

I am horrified to admit that I slept through Emmy's entire infamous pain lecture. I had so many questions, too.

I tried everything, honestly, I did. I fidgeted and squirmed and pinched myself and tried to take notes—nothing. I craved sleep in a way I have never known.

Once I accepted the fact that I would not stay awake, I spent at least 30 minutes plotting my escape. I'd slink down the hallway to the smaller creamsicle-colored yoga classroom. They have folding chairs in that room—so I'd set up the chairs and then drape sweaty yoga mats over the chairs—that's how they air them out. Only I'd use about six mats in a row, so it'd be like a tent and then I'd sleep under the tent. It would be the perfect place to hide and snooze.

I figured I'd at least stretch a little to keep my eyes from closing and look like, hey, I'm not asleep, I'm just stretching, keeping limber, I mean, it is a yoga college after all.

Put my legs in front of me, diamond-shaped, with the soles of my feet touching each other. I've always liked how that feels on the inside of my thighs, but I've never been able to bend forward too much.

Somehow, I dozed off in that position. When I woke up, I had my forehead on the ground. I had a toenail print on my cheek. Mind-body indeedy! When asleep—I'm limber as the next gal. Maybe I'm secretly as limber as Matmate Emily or Pigtail Sarah.

Yawning, Pudge Monkey reminds me that thin people are limber and Aunt Katherine was not limber and that I have to watch every bite.

WEDNESDAY 20 APRIL

Rajashree taught our morning class. Her classes almost feel like an out-of-body experience. Like when you go on vacation and you are kicking back at some out-of-the-way restaurant and the chef's wife comes out and sits at your table and tells you some long and meandering story about a cousin of hers. And you are slightly feeling annoyed at how much time she's taking to tell the story but then you remind yourself that you are on vacation and are all for new experiences and so you sit back and listen to the story of the chef's wife's cousin's parrot. That's what a Rajashree class feels like.

Bikram taught the evening class.

I've been experimenting with different places in the room—so I'm still in the front line, but five mats away from the podium. Funny—just switching to the right side of the podium and there are all these new faces I have never seen before. By switching around, I'm also hoping to blend a little.

Well, that, and, to be honest, I'm hoping to make friends.

A week ago, I was convinced roommate Yok was my officially-appointed Friend for Life. But she's been busy hanging with May, another girl from Thailand.

(Funny, though, she wanted to really get to know all the Asian teacher trainees. One gal from Australia, Jude, said she felt more Australian than Asian. And Yok got a similar response from this guy, Egan. He seemed almost offended and said he wasn't Asian at all, he was, clearly, Canadian.)

Anyway, I feel like TeflonGal; seems like the friendship thing isn't sticking. So many other people have already paired up, holding hands and hugging and whispering to each other during lunch. I feel really excluded and the part that baffles me is that we all came together as strangers, right? I mean, when I was The New Girl in school as we moved around, that's one kind of impenetrable bubble—kids who have been in kindergarten on up together.

I did have expectations that with everyone being The New Kid in school, it would be my one chance in four decades to just fit right in. Fit in, shop for Friend for Life. But after two weeks, the prognosis is a little bleak.

We get to Awkward, Bikram looks me in the eye and says, "Miss Pink, you have to get off your bar stool. You must sit down like the rest of the class. Second set, the entire class will wait for Miss Pink to get her ass off her bar stool."

Oh god.

I've got wicked bad knee pain. Bad knees. Knee surgery 23 years ago. And about two years ago, it seemed as though the surgery had run its course and the knees started creaking and hurting all over again.

I've spent this past year of yoga slowly getting down in the first part of Awkward and I'm all the way down in the third part of Awkward.

But the second part, up on your toes, balancing on the big toe, it just kills me. Plus which, some teachers have said that if your heels start to wobble, you shouldn't sit down any further, so I haven't, turns out my heels are quite wobbly indeed.

Bikram reminds me of the snake in Jungle Book. The eyes bewitch you and no matter how far away you are from the podium, when he calls you to do his bidding, it feels as though he's breathing his force into your nostrils. I swear I can feel the heat of his chai breath on my forehead.

I think I don't have a choice. I mean, I could say "no thanks" but I don't think that would go over well. Plus which, he's thrown down the gauntlet. The entire class will wait for me to sit down. Fine. They can wait then.

Our eyes lock on each other as I begin my descent. It feels as though we are two cowboys at sunset. We've agreed to the duel, the sun is setting and the saloon owner is taking bets on who will walk away alive.

UTKATASANA
AWKWARD

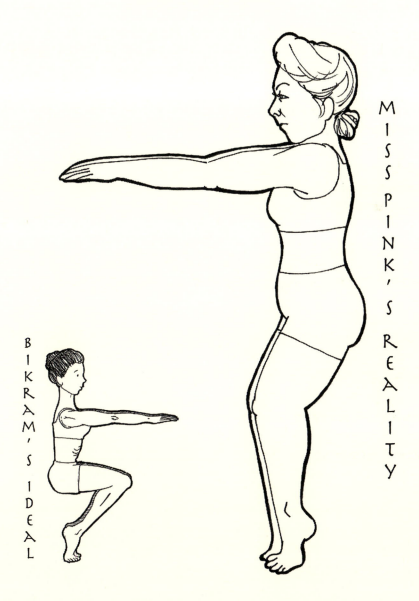

BIKRAM'S IDEAL

MISS PINK'S REALITY

I realized that this situation was the solution to my unrelenting fatigue.

I'm fairly certain that my kneecaps will crack in half as I heed his bidding. Once the kneecaps crack, Audrey Hepburn at the front desk will have to call an ambulance.

Once the ambulance gets here, the paramedics will have to throw open the wide side doors to the giant mirrored torture chamber. Once they do that, the room will cool down. So that's a big plus.

Once they've fetched me, they'll have to take me to an emergency room and emergency rooms are always well-cooled and, as an added bonus, I'll be able to sneak in a nap on the way.

Once I'm in the emergency room, some kind nurse will start a morphine drip, and then I'll sleep deeply and they will swaddle me in warm blankets.

All in all—pain relief, heat relief, and a giant 20-hour nap—what's not to like?

I've got tears making little splishy puddles in my lower eyelids. I feel I'm sitting down right to where the kneecaps will implode—and then—whooosh. A giant rush of no-pain sweeping through me. Almost like I had my own IV pole shooting white cold happy drugs straight into my veins.

The knees almost feel brand new, in an odd way.

The rest of the class, especially the floor series, presented some mental challenges.

There's this really nice girl next to me, Dana. Dark hair and funny and from Connecticut. We had talked earlier, doing the "Do you know Bob from Trumball?" kind of thing.

First off, she's quite bendy and so that makes me feel sort of less bendy. Or, like, you know, round Mento, skinny TicTac. I mean, if I were practicing next to my father, I'd like look like a goddess. But next to DarkHairDana—I think I'm just pale and blobby and I hate that Pudge Monkey is emboldened by this.

(Note to self: ask Dana about hair care products. She has zero split ends.)

We get to the floor series and she really has her arms stretched out quite wide. Which is okay, to each his own, etc. Except that apparently my mat was in her arm's way, so she actually pushed my left hand out of the way so she could have space on my mat. I mean, I think that's screwy, isn't it? Each person's mat is their own little playground, right?

So she keeps pushing my hand out of the way and then I'm thinking, well, what the hell is the etiquette? "Psst! Hey. Inner peace and all that rot, but get the wuck off my mat. Namaste."

Meanwhile, JauntyHatJaimie is two mats over and back and I keep thinking I should say something friendly to her. Though not sure what. Definitely would need to avoid hat chats and for sure not a peep about that whole Dr. Lilly thing. Then again, maybe it is best if I stay over on the left side of the room.

Plus which, Matmate Emily is comforting in an unspoken kind of way. An indescribable kind of way.

Interesting wrinkle tonight during Dialogue demos in front of Craig.

There's a guy, Andrew, who Yok has befriended.

So Yok has been on a mission to make friends with all the Asian students. I'll admit I feel sort of peevish—I mean, I've got to check off the Friends for Life box and I did think a roommate would be a slam dunk. Plus which, I lived in Taiwan as a child, so you'd think that would count for something.

Anyway, she immediately, duck-to-water, took to this Welshman named Andrew. He's included in her circle as he has married a Thai girl and lives in Bangkok.

At first, I think we were all a little taken with him. He seemed sort of clumsy yet affable, the way a puppy is cute when their waggy tail accidentally overturns the garbage pail. Turns out he is brain damaged. Was in an accident 15 years ago, smooshed spine, coma, the whole 9 yards. I tried to help him last week with the Dialogue, but he had an odd speech pattern that seemed unbreakable. He'd start strong and say about six words with conviction and then his words tumbled out of his mouth pellmell, like kids somersaulting down a hill.

Today, it was Andrew's turn to get up and deliver the Dialogue for Hands to Feet Pose.

Yok convinced May to come up and demonstrate as students for Andrew, so he'd have moral support.

Andrew got the first few sentences out with conviction and then the pellmell part of his brain took over and he stood there for a while, looking confused. I think the entire room had our collective fingers crossed for the chap.

Craig was prompting him, cuing him with bits of Dialogue to restart Andrew's engine.

Andrew said that he thought maybe he was on the wrong side of the students.

All us audience members looked at each other in confusion. Confusion turned to dropped jaws as he walked around behind the three lovely ladies and looked lasciviously at their rumps. To me, I got the sense of a drunk accountant at his first outing to a strip club.

Craig asked him what he was doing and he murmured something that sounded like, "I like Thai ass." Ripples of shock flitted through the room and lots of murmurs and whispers.

"What did he say?"

"Did he say Thai ass?"

"No, no, I think he said lemon grass."

"No, that doesn't fit. I think he meant chai glass."

"What's a chai glass? Some kind of drink?"

"Is that the sweet man who was in the accident?"

As we are registering this—he then says with a chuckle—"I think she do this wrong"—and proceeds to go up and touch the rump of one of the students.

Craig immediately brings everything to a screeching halt.

Sometimes things aren't what they seem.

THURSDAY 21 APRIL

# of days in yoga boot camp: 11

Woke up to stiff knees this morning—stiff, but also entirely without pain. However, decide I have to seek help for my bleeding feet.

Ever since that Saturday class when Craig said we couldn't drink water, and I was able to lick my knee cap, I realized that I can get my forehead to my knee in Standing Head to Knee—just have to put my mind to it.

This morning during Emmy's class, I have my forehead on my knee and my eyes are still focused down on the floor. I see red spots by my big toe and then I refocus my eyes and I see the red spots are blood. Ack! That's my blood dripping from my foot. I fall out and I'm so glad Emmy is nowhere in site.

Emmy tends to teach from the back of the room and she also tends to wander around. So you think you are safe and then you turn and then, blam!, she's right there, staring at you.

The gaze she shoots out is one of steely determination. I do honestly think that if any one person could single-handedly stop stupid war atrocities, it would be Emmy. I imagine her walking into Hussein's palace and saying, "Just stop it, Saddam. Enough already."

And she would intentionally mispronounce his name. If you place the emphasis on the second syllable and say sah-DAWM, you are saying, "Oh wise learned one."

However, Emmy would be smarter than that. If you drawl out the first syllable (thinking Bush #1 here) and say SAH-dem, you are saying, "little shoeshine boy."

So Emmy would know all that and in a crisp navy business suit and snappy heels, she'd walk through the palace and say "Enough already." Her voice simultaneously husky and crisp. He'd look into those eyes of hers and know she meant business.

It occurs to me that Emmy could moonlight for the U.S. government, if only they'd invent a Minister of War Stoppage. Because it should just be one person. I think that wars go on and on because no one is really sure which form to fill out to make it stop or which person gets the canary yellow copy of the form. With a Minister of War Stoppage, life would be a lot more fun and a lot less sad.

So, I've had these calluses on the tops of my feet, most likely from Fixed Firm Pose.

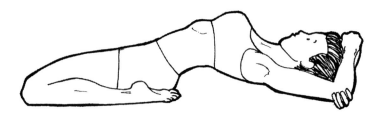

At first, I was really annoyed at the dark brown round spots on my feet. But once the calluses were well-established, my feet stopped hurting during Fixed Firm and I came to appreciate their role.

So then, the source of the dripping blood was exactly that—the calluses on both feet had hardened to the point that they were now split open.

I tried to think that this was a good development. During Standing Bow, the left foot split wide open. Roommate Yok and I decided it was a good sign—I was finally kicking hard enough to split open skin. (Lack of Friend for Life thing aside, I couldn't have asked for a more perfect roommate.)

I asked Craig and he looked down at my ucky feet and then looked at me as though he were running an ice cream store and feet issues were wholly unrelated to his universe. He said, "Hmm. Healing crisis," and nodded firmly, putting a period at the end of our sentence.

I asked Audrey Hepburn at the front desk and she said "Keep them clean."

We've had this great guest teacher visiting, Joel from Philadelphia. He just looks kindly and I went up to him after the evening class and he looked slightly alarmed. He asks if I've done band-aids. Who has time to buy band-aids? Suddenly I feel like an idiot—of course, band-aids! Joel also recommended sesame oil.

Yok, however, is concerned that sesame oil will be too stinky for foot application. And/or the sesame smell will cause unwanted hunger pangs in the middle of class.

Strawberry Julie agreed with Yok —having them split during Standing Bow is definitely a sign of strength.

FRIDAY 22 APRIL

# of days in yoga boot camp: 12

I really miss Prince. I miss him down to my toenails. If I were less tired and less temperature-freaky, I'd cry myself to sleep.

My thighs get white-hot at night and then turn to icicles. And when I wake up they are hot again but the center of my rump is frosty. Fellow teacher trainee Kay said, "Well, sounds like menopause." No! No! Not yet! "Well, perimenopause," Kay counters, sniffing my shock.

Kay's my hero. She's a standup comic and has naturally curly hair—and she's a four-year breast cancer survivor. And! when she was done with chemo she was diagnosed with Grave's disease.

Nonetheless, she's got a lot of moxie telling me menopause. A., I'm too young and B., who wants to hear that, casually, standing in line for a shower?

Redhead Amy overhears this and smirks. I do like her freckly face; she just looks both fun and warm. Amy is coming off a long relationship and struggling with her sense of self. She says she has so much pressure from her family. I tell her to screw the family—she has to follow her own heart's pathway. She gives me a funny glazed-over look.

I tell her I just have to disagree with the menopause diagnosis. I'm quite certain my hot/cold issues are entirely due to the apartment being so close to the ocean. Amy agrees heartily.

The fatigue is mostly gone by now—just one more class and the weekend is all mine.

Yok's husband Mike is in town for the weekend. It reminds me of summer camp; one kid gets a care package from mom and everyone gets homesick and cries.

As much as I can't fathom how I'd fit Prince into my jam-packed schedule, I see Yok light up like a Christmas tree and I envy her and I want my Prince to appear out of thin air.

SATURDAY 23 APRIL

# of days in yoga boot camp: 13

The 6:00 A.M. alarm comes too early, too fast. Time for yet another thigh-busting Craig class. This week Craig is a little sleepy (he's a self-proclaimed night owl)—though he terrorizes us in Awkward. We hold each segment over 60 seconds and I can no longer feel my left toes. They don't regain sensation until the floor series.

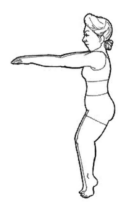

I am finally not weak-as-a-kitten on the floor. That's been the big battleground for me, oddly. Back at the Sweatbox, I felt tired during the standing series and then frisky and energized on the floor. Here, I feel like a bull through the balancing series and I want to weep when I get to the floor.

I feel large today. I say to Matmate Emily that I feel gi-normous. Emily says she thinks I've lost weight. Really? Honestly? Yes, yes, she assures me, she says she was talking with her van mates; they all thought I had been shrinking a bit. She's my new best friend and I will bake her brownies when I get home.

I whine to Yok that I feel heavy. Yok says, "You eat too much sugar. Try to not drink Vitamin Water and you won't feel fat."

I want to hit her. I resent it when skinny people jump in with boffo ideas on staying thin. May jumps in and says she read that if you put lemon juice in your water, you will lose weight.

Uh-huh. Nice. I look at both them with pursed lips. They burst into Thai and I feel left out. I am also slightly convinced they are saying, "She'll always be fat. Wonder if she'll fall for that lemon juice trick?"

I don't know why I am irritable, I just am. I buy People magazine and partake in a nice long Epsom salt bath and realize Yok is right; I have been socking away the Vitamin Water at an alarming rate. I'm just always so thirsty and they told us at the beginning to stay ahead of the thirst and could you really go wrong with water that has vitamins in it?

SUNDAY 24 APRIL

Off to cocktail party. Don't have a thing to wear. Bikram is hosting a fundraiser for Antonio Villaraigosa, some dude running for mayor of Los Angeles. Lots of folks grousing about having to go back into the big hot room on our one day off. I don't mind; I think it'll be fun to see what people look like in regular clothing.

Meanwhile, yoga drama has hit home in the form of brain-injured Andrew.

Andrew had come to our apartment yesterday, ringing the doorbell, wanting Narina. I have never heard that name before and I tell him he's got the wrong place and he looks like he's going to cry.

I close the door and a few minutes later, he's ringing the bell again. He found the piece of paper Narina gave to him. He gives it to me like it is a claim ticket and I'll surely just turn around and hand him his hat.

Close the door, ding-dong, no Narina, lather rinse repeat.

Today, I'm talking with my mum on the phone and there he is again, at the door. I say he must be confused, this is where Yok lives. He says "Yok who?" and I feel slightly mad and slightly sorry for Yok. She's actually helped him do laundry a couple of times this past week.

Andrew gets really angry and when I close the door, he loses his temper, he's banging on the door and he so very much wants me to let him in, he knows Narina is hiding from him. He also says, "I remember now, Yok, she will let me in."

I feel a little vulnerable. Yok and Mike are out shopping and our upstairs neighbors are out by the pool and this Andrew guy is physically in great shape and quite strong. Nonetheless, that's what chains on doors are for.

Besides which, just because he's brain damaged doesn't mean he's nice. I repeat this over and over, a mantra, a way of making sure I don't give in to his puppy dog brown eyes and big floppy feet.

I walk away from the front door and loudly close my bedroom door—and he stands there, banging.

Five minutes of silence, followed by more fist-banging on my door, more mewling. It feels straight out of Streetcar Named Desire, right down to the white tank top. He's yelling at the top of his lungs. Narina and Yok stole from him. They stole his money. He wants his money. They put the money under the bed. He must come in and go under the bed to get his money.

Yok comes home from shopping right as he's given up his post and they talk in the hallway, her and Andrew. I tell her he's not well and she laughs and says its okay, he is nice, he's just not all there.

Maybe I am being overly-jeebed? Then again, I survived living across from the housing projects in Brooklyn's infamous Bedford-Stuyvesant neighborhood—and I wasn't ever this unnerved.

Yok agrees to go with Andrew to help him. I implore her husband, Mike, to at least go with her. He laughs it off in a jolly kind of way, no, no she'll be fine.

Yok returns about 30 minutes later. I didn't think she had it in her to be that mad.

Turns out she had, with her big giant heart, given Andrew a phone card so he could call his wife in Thailand. He tried to use the card to call his mum in Wales and it wouldn't work—it was just for Thailand. She tried to explain it to him and he ramped back up into sheer anger and he threw the card at her. She lost her Thai sweetness and yelled that she didn't have to be nice to him and she couldn't believe what a butt head he had become.

She's relaying this story to me and all I can think of is: what a great voice. We've talked about how when she talks in Thai with May her voice is powerful and commanding. And when she switches to English, her voice is very small and timid. So for the past week or so, I've been trying to help her find her teacher's voice.

There it is. Mid-rant, I interrupt her and I say, "That's it! That's your teacher's voice."

She looks like she'd throw daggers at me if she could and I said, "Say the first paragraph of Half Moon," and she does and it is phenomenal.

She agrees (finally)—he's a scary man, Andrew. We decide we will take the issue up with Craig tomorrow—neither of us feel very safe at this point.

Meanwhile, I must must shower and clean up and look halfway normal for this soiree.

Yok keeps coming into my room asking when I'm leaving. Every 20 minutes, I'm sitting here, writing like mad, and then, blam, the creative merry-go-round grinds to a halt with her sweet little Thai voice calling out, "You are going to be late, you know."

I'm about to go out there and tell her to piss off. And then it dawns on me. With a bit of a forehead smack, I realize that perhaps she and hubby want some time alone.

Have I mentioned? I miss Prince so much my throat hurts.

MONDAY 25 APRIL

# of days in yoga boot camp: 15

Yok and I decide we will keep to our resolve and talk to Craig about the Andrew situation. I confide to Matmate Emily and she, too, had been having issues with him. She agrees to speak with Craig as well.

We both still feel a little jittery though, Yok and I. Her husband Mike remains very laissez faire and that chafes me. Mostly because it reminds me of Prior Husband and how often he shrugged at things that were important to me.

I put my mat down for the morning class, go back outside to fix my hair. When I come back to my mat, I find that Andrew is two spots over.

Damnit. I can't move now, it would be awfully obvious and it might hurt his feelings. But it is my neighborhood, these are my peeps and I've never seen Andrew on this side of the room before. (Emily is no where to be found, though.)

Besides which, at 9:25, all the good spots are taken.

We make eye contact. Andrew says, with his sweet puppy voice, "Sorry I was an asshole."

I thought, okay, great, nice of him to apologize. I said, "You know, you really scared me Andrew."

He rises up off his elbows and says, "No I didn't."

We do an absurd did not/did too volley. I tried to bring it to an end by asking that he not bang on my door again.

He furrowed his innocent-looking eyebrows and said, "But I had to bang on the door; Yok stole money from me."

Whatever hesitations I had about talking with Craig—vanished like a mist into the room.

I also found out from Yok that the mystery "Narina" Andrew sought was none other than Yok's friend May. Narina is her given Thai name but she prefers to go by May.

For reasons not entirely clear, May apparently invited Andrew to visit her in our apartment, which is just hinky 16 ways under. I try to talk to May about this and she gets blinky and teary and says I wouldn't understand.

I remember Craig telling us to stay out of yoga drama, so I drop the thread.

Bikram taught the Monday night class. I did move my mat over five spaces and back one row, hoping to hide from Bikram. I was just a little freaky about the Andrew thing and my knees were pretty stiff.

Sure 'nuff, in Awkward Pose, Bikram is staring at me. He says nothing. Instead, he points his finger down to the ground and I know, I know, I need to sit down more. I nod and smile at him, I'm so happy he has let me be.

In the second set of Awkward, he says "Miss Pink!" I almost burst into tears, I think, oh no, no, no, I cannot withstand a withering blast from you nor can my knees. I look at him quickly, hoping to convey my pitiful state to him.

He got it. His face softened a little and he said, "Good Miss Pink. NOW you lean back lean back lean back lean back lean back." I was so happy he asked for something I could actually do.

After dinner, I went in to talk to Craig about my own yoga drama. I was slightly concerned that Craig had fallen under Andrew's spell and feared an uphill slog.

Craig was really very, very nice about the whole thing. He asked if I was okay and strongly encouraged me to call the police the next time someone bangs on my door. Wanted to know if there was anything, anything at all, that they could do for me. I just said I was concerned that with his brain injury, it appears that Andrew has impulse control issues. I did admit I was afraid he'd get mad if he perceived I was 'turning him in.' Craig said there had already been some discussions about the issues he was having with the training.

Craig also stressed that I needed to be ready to go in and talk to Bikram directly. He said it could be unnerving, talking with the king. I smiled a tired little smile and said, why no, speaking with Bikram would be fine.

TUESDAY 26 APRIL

# of days in yoga boot camp: 16

Craig did warn us. He did say to watch out for the "yoga truck." The truck runs over you and sometimes hits reverse and backs over you and flattens you. You are under duress, you are sweating profusely three hours a day, you must cram for anatomy tests, you don't get enough sleep, your chakras open, muscle tissues cough up memories, you weep, you laugh, you weep while laughing.

I'm not quite under the truck's wheels just yet—but I do feel like I can hear the noisy diesel engine rattling right outside my window.

We have heard no word on Andrew. Yok and I (and to some extent Emily) are wound pretty tightly. We are also convinced people are looking at us funny. No doubt there's some kind of gossip flowing through the grapevine. Andrew is not there for the morning class and he did not sign in for class either. Again, Tuesday night's class, there's still no sign of him. This elusiveness puts more smelly diesel in my idling yoga truck, I feel it in my shoulders, my clavicle feels torqued.

For reasons I can't explain, I keep thinking about my third date with my Prince. And how I just knew on that day, I knew we were destined to be together. That was the first time he proposed, on date number three. I played coy, but secretly, I was dancing a jig. Even now, six months into our glorious marriage, I still haven't told him that I knew I'd say yes on that day.

Emmy teaches the morning class and kicks our ass in her usual way. Sweet there-there grandma cooing. Next thing you know, she's got us in Balancing Stick for, I swear to Ganesh, minutes on end, talking about opening up chakras and chicken slaughter techniques and you think your heart will pop and a lung will implode and she's prattling and prattling.

In the middle of our endless Balancing Stick, it dawned on me that I really wanted O-U-T out. I was tired and I wanted to nap right then and there. I mean, I don't think there's a rule against that. They frown upon leaving the room or sticking your nose under the door crack to huff fresh air, but no one has specifically said, "no napping during class."

I find myself asking what the hell am I doing here? What am I trying to prove? I mean, what's with the heat? Seriously—do we have any scientific proof it should always be this hot?

Maybe I'd have just as much fun doing yoga in 68 degrees, in a turtleneck, supping cocoa and serving gluten-free brownies during savasana. Right? Right.

And I'm mad and frustrated and people are leaving the room en masse. Sort of like how you always see clumps of people in a mass exodus, they are always clumped up. Moral support, I suppose. There are bunches of three, four, five people just nodding at each other and getting up and leaving. I'm feeling left out, and I wonder if they have all already made their Friend for Life. I'm envisioning the mango smoothies they are sipping in the hallway and if I weren't in the first row, I'd run screaming from the inferno.

Even Firefighter Charlie leaves the room. Damnit! That really did me in. I mean, the guy used to run into glowing, toasty buildings for a living. If the firefighter thinks it is too hot, I think we should all leave.

Morality Monkey shrieks the loudest; he is dismayed to think I would go back on my goals. Pudge Monkey is pretty listless, but manages to convince me that if I weren't so fat, I wouldn't be so hot.

Craig talks at length after dinner about choosing to do Bikram Yoga and choosing to come to training. He says we should not beat up on ourselves, we need to realize that what we are embarking on takes courage and that we are an incredible group of courageous people.

The word courage makes me cry. For 10 minutes during lecture, the tears just run down my face.

Allie—a free spirited let's-skinnydip-in-the-moonlight type—looks at my tears and says, "Aww, the yoga truck?" and I nod. I fear a hug, it will make me wail like a wounded dog, the way Becky the poodle wailed that one time her paw got stuck under a door. Allie rubs my toes and comments on how cool it is that I have triangle toes.

I burbled into the phone Tuesday night to Prince, I cry, I shouldn't, I should be brave but I can't, I miss him and I miss how he cooks salmon and I miss our salads with goat cheese and cranberries and why, oh why, did I think I could go five weeks without seeing him?

I feel better, though, after crying into the phone. I have a nipper of chocolate and decide that I'm over the yoga truck thing after all. Wasn't too bad, actually.

WEDNESDAY 27 APRIL

# of days in yoga boot camp: 17
# of days until I see Prince: 23

Go into the room this morning and it was reallyreallywuckinghot. The goal for a standard Bikram Yoga class is a temperature of about 105 degrees with humidity around 50 percent. I don't mind the drippiness, I really don't. In fact, I usually look at all the sweat running off me as good—I've got it to sweat out, thank god it found the exit door.

Dry heat though, the kind that makes your nostril hairs hurt, dry heat I just abhor.

And that was this morning. Dry and insanely hot. It seemed like I had to fight the urge to leave every seven seconds.

Here's how I imagined my exit: I'd hear a taxi pull up outside. I'd know it was a taxi because taxi brakes always squeal, almost like they are whining, "Don't stop here. Not heeeerrre." And then taxi's door would slam hard. The current passenger stands by the side of the idling taxi and sorts out the singles in the wallet. The passenger would walk into Bikram's World Headquarters and the driver would pull out his clipboard and make notes.

That's when I simply turn and briskly walk out of the room. I'd have a determined look on my face, a look that says, "Darn it! I just remembered. I need to be at my dentist's office in 10 minutes. Summer bleaching, you know." I'd even look at my watch to emphasize the point that I have an appointment and I'm running late.

I won't stop for anything. No shoes, no water, no wallet. I simply stride with my head held high and I get into the taxi and I say, "The airport please." Actually, no, I'd ask that he first take me across the street to the fitness place to get a pineapple smoothie and then we'd go to the airport and I'd walk up to the ticketing agent and explain my predicament. As luck would have it, the agent does Bikram Yoga and is a friend of Rajashree's, and I get a boarding pass and then I get on the airplane and the stewardess says, "Can I get you anything?" and I ask for a blanket and I sleep and when I wake up, Prince is waiting for me at the airport.

I believe I spent about 75 percent of class planning my taxi exit. A little planning would help. For example, if I put my wallet in my shoes by the door—then I'd be successful in my plan. The taxi driver would surely demand payment (especially for the smoothie) and then, realistically, you simply cannot get on an airplane without a photo ID, no matter the situation.

I don't think this is a good sign, the exit-route planning. I'm quite certain that Emily and Leo and Strawberry Julie are all standing there thinking "I love this yoga! I love this heat! I'm so glad I'm not chubby like that girl in pink over there!"

Usually timid and soft-spoken, Morality Monkey is having a fit, he just cannot believe how seriously I'm considering leaving. He thought we had this all worked out yesterday. He throws down the gauntlet and calls me a coward.

I'm pretty sure I'm not a coward. Heck, I've made it this far, maybe that's my path, to have tried it and then said, "Nah, no thanks, this is not my cup of tea."

(Speaking of tea—I still cannot find Oregon Chai and I'm quite low.)

Many students—including Matmate Emily—have been spending time in the steam room, which is about 187 degrees with small rain clouds in the corners. I've been muttering "heat freaks" under my breath every time I walk by. Steam room fans claim that after 187 degrees, 105 degrees feels downright like a frisky fall day.

Emily seems nice and sane, so I wade into the fairly crowded steam room and I can't take that heat either, I feel sick, I want my mommy, I want my kitten, I want my tea, and then a popsicle. I can't find Emily through the soupy fog, so I plunk down on the bench. Next to me is Kelly, an exceedingly perky professional dancer that can put her toes above her head just for fun. I don't know her well, but I'm glad it is her. I need—well—I need help.

I turn to Kelly and I say, "I don't think I can do it today. The room, today, you know, was umm, you know, kind of, um, extra hot."

I feel like a fool. All this time, 17 long days in yoga boot camp, and you never hear anyone talking directly about the heat. It just isn't done.

Kelly laughs and tosses her bouncy Shirley Temple curls (even her hair is perky!) and says, "Yah. Totally hot. Don't worry, you'll do it. I know you can." And then she spritzed us with eucalyptus. And I cried, but just a wee bit.

I made it through class, one minute at a time. The eucalyptus spray was strong and stayed on my forearms and shoulders. Every time I had the vision of my taxi exit, I'd sniff my forearms and smell the eucalyptus and think, "A complete stranger believes in me."

On the Andrew front: he is gone. He has vanished without a trace. Bikram folks went to his apartment late Tuesday and it is utterly empty. Gone without a trace, fridge immaculate.

I find the fridge thing extra creepy. Who packs up and goes home—all the way back to Bangkok no less—in 18 hours? And cleans the fridge?

Almost to the weekend. Prince says a surprise will arrive Friday night—I'm hoping it is my damn tea. I miss my morning ritual, my chai. I gave up coffee (quite begrudgingly) last year and found this great chai that really hits the spot. I've been rationing it out, having a little cup in the evening, the perfect compliment to gluten-free brownies baked and sent to me by my friend Stewart.

THURSDAY 28 APRIL

# of days in yoga boot camp: 18
# of days until I see Prince: 22

I feel mentally a little cheerier today but physically kind of off.

My feet have stopped bleeding, so that's progress.

However, I'm having chest pains, which is probably not a good sign any way you slice it. Right at the sternum, under the left breast area. Heart attack? Tumor growth? Too many veggies for lunch?

The good news is that it really hurts when I push on it, so that rules out mammogram concerns. Mum always reminds me at mammogram time, "Remember, that's why they call cancer the silent killer. It doesn't hurt at all."

Bikram decides tonight is the night to explain to us the history of yoga. I can't wait—there's so much I don't know. I took copious and thorough notes, mostly to stay awake.

Here's the History of Yoga.

This woman is in the kitchen and realizes her dinner recipe calls for monkey lips. She asks her husband to be a sweetheart and go get monkey lips. Husband gets out there and realizes he doesn't know what kind of monkey or how many monkeys. So he picks up an entire mountain and moves the mountain to outside the wife's kitchen window. That is how strong the gods are, they move mountains. Americans are not strong at all, they can put a man on the moon but they are incapable of putting their damn toes on the line.

(Bikram has blue lines on the carpet, as he likes us lined up in a row. Pet peeve of his.)

I think I missed something, but from the astronauts we return to the creation of yoga. One yogi created three beings from lotus bloom out of his navel. There are eight brothers and they decide to play a prank and they steal a cow.

(I'm not certain, but I think maybe they stole the cow of one of the belly button blooming yogi people.)

God gets quite mad and sends all eight brothers down to earth, to live as humans. God tells them to meditate. They complain, they simply cannot sit and meditate for a lifetime, their rumps hurt, they have to go to the bathroom (I imagine they'd get kind of hungry, too, along the way). God tells them tough nuggies, they should not have stolen the cow of the bellybutton person. They begin to move in different ways and those movements become postures and that is yoga. The end.

FRIDAY 29 APRIL

# of days in yoga boot camp: 19
# of days until I see Prince: 21

Morning class is a tough one taught by Rajashree. I didn't entirely entertain any exit fantasies but I did spend some time wondering why I am chubby. I mean, I count my calories and, here I am, exercising hours a day and I'm still kind of chubby looking. I look at Rajashree a lot during class and she's a normal looking person, she's not a toothpick, she looks just right. I have an overwhelming desire to know what she weighs. Like I think that if I could look as pretty as Rajashree, then my monkeys would sleep and I'd have some quiet time with myself.

We are going at a good pace with the Dialogue; that's what they tell us. We are at the balancing series. Standing Head to Knee.

They have also broken us up into six small groups; I am in group 2. I do scan my group and I'm not getting any kind of Friend for Life vibe at all.

Since we are in smaller groups, we need lots of people to be behind the clipboard now. Teachers from prior trainings come back each year to help with learning the Dialogue. I think that's just amazing – isn't it?

I muff my Dialogue a little in the afternoon. I miss two sentences, which tweaks me, but my improvisational skills kick in and I keep words coming out of my mouth. Funny, I've been struggling with the posture so much in class—I wonder how much of that is carrying over into my vocal delivery of the accompanying Dialogue.

You know what it is? I mean, this is almost mortifying, but I fear mediocrity. Usually when I do something, I excel, I'm out of this world. Like the time I went to volunteer at the kayaking Olympic trials and I was supposed to serve coffee and sign people in, and then I got promoted to gate judge, and then I got promoted to area judge, which was awesome, sitting on a rock in the middle of a snake-infested river, deciding who cleared the gate and who didn't.

Or when I worked on the trading desk. I didn't wake up one day and say to myself, "I know, I'm awful at math and fractions confuse me—I know—I'll face those fears head-on in the heart of Wall Street."

No, I was down to $98 in my checking account and was already 1 month behind on rent and I took a temp job as a secretary and then someone said I wrote well, I could make sense of things and so then I got promoted to note-taker and then 6 months later, I'm on the trading desk with 300 sweaty men.

Here—I feel like I'm at the bottom of the food chain. I'm probably the only student in the room plotting my escape and I'm probably the only person in the room that has cross-dressing monkeys running around in her brain. And in a couple of postures—we are going into uncharted waters—the second half of the Dialogue that I haven't even looked at and so once we are into that deep, dark, scary area, I fear this will turn into The One Thing I Really Suck At.

Which really stinks because it won't be a private moment, the sucking. You know, it isn't like I tried to take up knitting in the comfort of my nonheated living room and I was awful at it and then I tossed the knitting needles in the junk drawer with old keys and leftover chopsticks and no one is wiser. No, this will be a public downfall and I dread it.

During anatomy class (which usually runs from noon until around 3:00) about half of the students were fast-asleep. I was really battling the heavy eyelids, too, and may have dozed off here and there. Up until today, I've been fairly awake—not necessarily alert, but at least my eyes are open. But as I listened to little tiny snores from all over the room, I decided I had nothing to prove, who am I to stay awake when everyone else sleeps?

All of the sudden, the big doors to the studio are thrown open and it is Bikram. He yells like an angry parent, a parent who found his kid in the liquor cabinet, he's so angry we are dozing.

At first I think he's going to have some kind of diva moment, some kind of "I am wrathful and in charge of your fate so everyone who snored will not graduate" kind of thing.

Doors wide open, he's yelling. Then he says, "You all need a break. You cannot sit for hours and hours. Move! Get up! Come see my new car." Not just any car, but a brand-new Bentley.

(Rumor has it he owns 85 cars; then again, I've also heard whispers that he has 85 Rolex watches.)

He's like a kid on Easter Sunday, he's found the best Easter egg and he can't wait to show it off. He seems pretty fine letting 200 sweaty half-asleep yogis play in his new car.

Money Monkey runs the numbers. Bentleys usually are priced in the $200,000 range. So what is the car payment on this new car? Close to $1600/month? Is that right? And then if he really does own 85 Bentleys, that would imply $100,000/month on car payments alone?

***

Talked with Redhead Amy in the garage during break time. She spends her break time reading the New York Times in her car. Says she likes being a bit by herself. Hmm. Kept wondering if she was trying to hint that I needed to step away from her car, but I'm hungry for a little conversation.

We talk about her Prior guy and my Prior Husband and the similarities: depression, mood swings, cuddly and cute when sober. I even joke that perhaps we were with the same man. I promise her I'll bring in a copy of my manuscript, Leaving the Land of Should; I'm convinced it will cheer her right up.

**

The evening class is taught by a high-octane Bikram. I'm feeling a little wimpy, so I move bravely into the third row and I don't wear pink. I'm head-to-toe navy. Not that I can hide from the man, but a little camouflage can't hurt.

I swear, he has some kind of magical eyes. There I am, in blue, in the third row, minding my own business, feeling acky in Hands to Feet.

Booming over the microphone, his dulcet tones. "Miss Pink. Lock your knees now."

Probably not me. Lots of other pink outfits in the room. No sense in locking now, I can't spend all my energy right here in the second posture, can I?

"Yes, you. Miss Pink, I talk to you, you think you can hide from me? You know my eyes. Now. Lock. Your. Knees."

Hmm. Maybe he is talking to me. Am I still Miss Pink? I'll do it halfway, I think to myself, just a smidge, so that if it is me, he'll see I'm trying and if it isn't me, then I haven't depleted my energy banks.

"No, Miss Pink, LOCK your knees, not halfway, all da way. Lock. Your. Damn. Knees. Miss. Pink."

Owie, owie, owie, I've snapped something, surely something is ruined, it hurts so bad that I've lost my urge to ack, which I guess is good, but I do so want to cry.

PADA HASTASANA
HANDS TO FEET

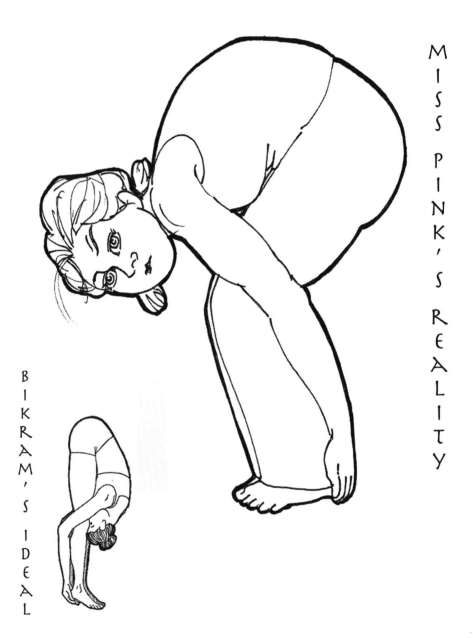

MISS PINK'S REALITY

BIKRAM'S IDEAL

"Better Miss Pink."

Nice surprise, in a way. My knees were locked for the first time ever in my life and it did hurt like hell. Then again, interesting to see what the body will do when the mind knows no other choice.

It was also a two-hour class, which explains why I ran out of water.

He's actually quite kind, I think. I mean, he didn't have to say "Better Miss Pink"—but that little pat on the back just kept me going, kept me floating the rest of the class.

The cherry on top is that Bikram gives us Friday night off—which is just fab—because— my surprise from Prince is him at the airport.

Hoooooorrrrah! What a prince. He was going to make it an uber-surprise (not tell me at all and sneak in late at night) but thought, what with all the Andrew excitement this week, that a stealth visitor late at night might provoke a different kind of excitement.

SUNDAY 1 MAY

# of days in yoga boot camp: 21

Had a great session with my chiropractor yesterday. Turns out I had two ribs out of place causing the wicked chest pain. Took some work, but we did get them back into place and the pain is gone. He also gave me an exercise to keep them in place in the future.

As quickly as he appeared, Prince vanished tonight. He'll be back in three weeks for my birthday. It doesn't seem too far away now that we've had an intermission.

Yok called Andrew. The rumors of his zippy exodus had refused to die down. In fact, the new twist is that he had stopped practicing yoga entirely and his old injuries had started to flare up again.

Yok had his phone number from all those times she helped him—so she and May talked with him and he's doing really well. She got the sense from him that he knew going into it that it was a long shot, his graduating. But he was glad he had tried and yes, he's still doing the yoga. He also told Yok that he didn't blame anyone for his return home—so as much as I wasn't sure she should call him, I'm glad to hear he is okay.

Hope this week gels better on mind and body feeling better. Big anatomy test tomorrow. Once that's out of my hair, it'll be a bit easier to focus on Dialogue, Dialogue, Dialogue.

MONDAY 2 MAY

# of days in yoga boot camp: 22
# of days until I see Prince: 18

The room is just obscenely, obnoxiously HOT. Stultifying. Claustrophobic. I put my mat down and immediately leave the room. To avoid the room until the last possible minute, I'm now oh-so happy to spend a little extra 'quality time' in the women's locker room. The locker room is about as packed as the #4 express train out of Grand Central at 6 P.M. on a Friday night.

One gal, Chasity, is having her own yoga truck moment.

Chasity fascinates me. She's the mother of 3 children, she looks like she's about 20 years old, she's from Las Vegas, and she says she's an exotic dancer. I'm desperate to ask her if that means exotic in the less-clothing category? And if so, I have about 97 questions about that. How did she start? Is she shy by nature? What does she tell her kids? What does she do on days she feels bloated and icky? Does she have to hide her income source from "mommy and me" groups?

She told me that with her first childbirth, she cracked her pelvis. No one knew it was cracked, they chalked up her discomfort to standard labor pains.

Somehow, she was talked into a second child, and the crack deepened. Then, with the third child, they did an X-ray and found the crack. Isn't that astonishing? I think it is. Then she does the yoga and the pain goes away.

Anyway, I'm hanging in the bathroom, avoiding the firey inferno, and Chasity is one unhappy camper. She's yelling that the room is just too damn hot. It isn't right. Something must be broken. She wants to go home. She has three kids for god's sake, she has never been away from her kids, she simply cannot go into that room.

Lots of people are looking out of the corner of their eyes and are slowly slinking away from her yoga truck. Not out of lack of compassion, but more a sense of self-preservation. At that moment, I realized I wasn't the only person wanting to run screaming from the room.

I told Chasity she'd come this far already and she'd always regret leaving at this point. For the love of god, she can give birth to children with a cracked pelvis, surely 90 minutes in a stinky hot room is less painful than that, right?

Plus which, we are in week #4 already! We are two days away from the official halfway point.

She's just staring at me as though I've offered her a plate of steaming tripe. Usually I've won over my audience by this point.

Desperate, I borrowed a line from Perky Kelly. "I know you can do it."

And then I walked away—I knew if I stayed longer, I'd tell her of my taxi exit and I still had my wallet in my hand and she'd probably talk me into leaving.

Got a great e-mail from Saiko, a teacher at the Sweatbox. Saiko is actually a key player in my yoga journey. My second class ever as a student was her first class ever as a teacher. She's Japanese with a singsong voice; in fact, she is now teaching Bikram classes in Japanese.

As I tried to pep talk myself into applying for Yoga College, I kept thinking of Saiko's courage. English isn't her first language, and yet, she wasn't daunted, she sucked it up, she made it through.

Saiko is also teensy—barely 5 feet tall, probably weighs 100 pounds with shoes on and wet hair. She has such a beautiful practice to boot.

Anyhoo, she wrote to say she was coming to LA to help with yoga boot camp. I whined to her (as I have to anyone that will listen) that I'm so bloated and that I feel huge. Saiko emailed right back and said she gained 10 pounds in the beginning of teacher training. I felt oddly relieved/happy about that. That's 10 percent weight gain, even in her, a teensy little thing. She promises the bloat does go away. I'll cling to that morsel of wisdom.

Craig scolds us for our water habits and encourages us to consider doing the class without water. I swear to god, he was trying to stare right into my well-hydrated eyes as he talked about this.

Freak. No water! That's just crazy talk. I mean, I'm all about training and doing things well, but when the room is a zillion degrees, there is simply no way Jose, am I giving up water.

I usually drink about 64 ounces of water during each class and I still end up losing 2 to 4 pounds after each class—nope, sorry, WeirdoBoy, nope, I must, must, must have the water.

I'm not sure if it was the no water talk, but I thought today that he looked a little less like Bull Durham Kevin Costner. I think he's as skanky-looking as Waterworld Costner.

TUESDAY 3 MAY

# of days in yoga boot camp: 23
# of days until I see Prince: 17

This morning's class was hotter than yesterday, if at all possible. I'm guessing at least 120 degrees and a gazillion percent humidity. I used to count the number of sweat drops coming off my body. Today, I counted the streams of water. During Eagle, I had three separate rivers of sweat just running in a solid stream—all from one arm. I did not have time to count the rivers pouring off my butt and foot.

How hot was it? It was sooooo hot that there was actually a line to get out the door. At one point, there were eight people on the left side of the room and six people on the right side, all just standing in line, waiting to get out the door. I'd estimate close to 40 people just upped and left.

I decide to try less water. I won't do no water, I just think there's a safety issue involved, I don't care that people in India do it without a mat and without water, I'm not in Calcutta, am I? No. I'm in the land of the free, which means freedom of the press, freedom of speech, freedom to slurp.

However, I'm also slightly worried that they'll make us do a water-free class, so I'd like to have some experience under my belt. One guy, Mike, does the class w/out any water at all—so he's cheering me on. I do leave my large water bottle at the back of the room, under the fire alarm, in case I need to run to it. And I did eke out two classes with just 10 ounces of water. Lots and lots of mind monkeys are shrieking in the trees, but I persevere.

There's a new guy in town, a teacher from Washington, DC, named Jim. He's a retired Army Airborne Ranger, which I think sounds quite zippy. He said he's done combat tours in Viet Nam and Desert Storm. That seems like quite a lot. Anyway, Jim is very very hard-core. It seems pretty unusual to go from the military into yoga – talk about opposite ends of the lifestyle spectrum. He does walk back and forth and sets his rules down for the posture clinic he'll be running. His crispness seems very much out of place here. Sort of like seeing neon glow sticks at the opera.

When Jim graded people on Dialogue, he spent about five minutes per person saying things like "On the fifth line, you missed the word nicely. And then on the fourteenth line, you missed chin up."

Bah and humph and feh.

I don't know why, but he reminds me of one of the guys from my lovely college marching band fiasco.

It is funny where life takes you. Two decades, and I twitch and quiver just thinking about the college marching band situation.

***

I come from a long line of marching band people. Mum and dad marched, as did my two aunts-all together in their high school band. My sister, too, marched in both high school and college.

I followed in their footsteps and marched in my high school band and was so anxious to march in the college band. I was so looking forward to it. I was to play the piccolo, which I love. Midsummer, the band director wrote to say that I'd also need to play saxophone from time to time.

My podium-throwing high school band director was, in fact, an alumnus of the college band and he volunteered to give me saxophone lessons throughout the summer.

What went completely unmentioned was that this particular band had a long tradition of being all-male. Since my name is one of those ambiguous boy/girl names, they just assumed that I was a guy, so there were some surprises at the beginning.

There was a lot of hazing. It started out all in fun: no bathing for a week, wear a beanie on your head, hold a match while reciting a poem, that sort of thing. It was an intense week, that first one, between the hazing and the marching. But, I was anxious to make this my new family, my new batch of friends. (Hmm. Shades of Friends for Life quest?)

Initiation week plunged us into new levels of depravity. Most of us were physically hassled throughout the week. Us pledglings, though, we stuck together and kept counting down the days until the first football game and then the formal initiation after the game. Even the governor flew in for the event—he, too, was a former band member.

After the game, we returned to the band hall. The band hall's usual chaos was gone. In its stead were rented chairs and a large table draped with cloth and lots of candles -- and all the seniors were wearing hooded outfits. Sort of like they bought Ku Klux Klan outfits at a tag sale and then dyed them black.

There was a lot of whiskey drinking. Then a branding iron came out and a fire was lit. Our membership into the band would be complete once the governor branded us with this dinner-plate sized logo and we drank the sacred horse blood.

I may have been a naive 18 year old, but it seemed like whiskey and flame was not a good combo. That, and the branding iron was quite large and I scar funny.

I raised my hand and said, "Umm. No thank you." And there was quite a hubbub and then two other pledglings said "No thank you" and then I was the rabble-rouser and the hooded seniors were displeased. The band elders decided that if I stayed late after the branding, I could atone for my sassiness and perform a few duties and still be initiated.

I was told I'd even have a choice in what duties I'd perform. My little mind monkeys were cheering, high-fiving each other. See, they said, see, don't judge hooded drunk men so quickly.

I opted for performing some kind of repulsive duty, like cleaning the vomit out of the tuba or scrubbing the frightening potty. I was surprised (understatement of the decade) when I was told option #1 involved being blindfolded and naked and allowing seniors to "have their way" with the 3rd female ever to join the band.

Suddenly, barfy brass instruments are looking pretty good.

Option #2 was to play the mystery pledge game. I quickly opted for mystery over nakedness.

The mystery game was called "Kaboom." It went like this: they'd throw a beer can on to the floor. I'd have to throw myself on that beer can, as it represented a land mine that would kill all the seniors and, as a pledge, it was my job to give up my life for the seniors. When the seniors yelled "kaboom," I had to make my body fly up into the air.

Levitation is not in my skill set. So they 'helped' me fly, picking me up by my arms and ankles and tossing me about like a rag doll.

The end result was many cracked ribs, one cracked kneecap, one displaced kneecap. When I went to the emergency room, the triage nurse said, "Oh, the band. Okay, we'll get the band doctor in." Apparently, the band members had done quite a lot of pledge injuring over the years, and had a well-oiled machine in place to take care of the damaged freshmen.

***

One way the memory of Kaboom pops up is in Awkward. Every time I push my limits and sit down further than I like, I feel the front of my kneecap throbbing, there's a quick flash of memory, fear, kaboom, pain. It hadn't really bothered me—we are who we are, individualized quilts of memories both good and bad. That and I had been avoiding sitting down more deeply to avoid the memory flash.

Sometimes I wonder—all those people that tossed my body about like a rag doll—are they having flashbacks too? Are they sitting in a restaurant, ordering a second round of garlic sticks, saying, "Speaking of garlic, Hon, did I ever tell you about the time in college, that one girl I threw against the wall?"

WEDNESDAY 4 MAY

# of days in yoga boot camp: 24
# of days until I see Prince: 16

Rajashree taught the morning class. Not as stupid hot as before, but a challenge nonetheless. I am okay with dribbles of water and only sup every 25 minutes or so. I've gone from 60+ ounces per class down to about 10 ounces per class and, I've got to admit, I do feel more energetic.

I'm a little worried about the Dialogue. I haven't really gotten posture #7, Balancing Stick nailed down. Craig heard my last bit of Dialogue and said that if I stop ad-libbing and say the words exactly, then he'll let me "run wild."

Balancing Stick is mentally taxing—you have to convince yourself that of course you can stand on one leg and balance there, your body a letter T-like-Tom from the side.

All the instructors (except for Jim the military Dialogue freak) are encouraging people to ad-lib a little. When you are balancing on one leg and the heart is pounding, you do need some rah-rah-ing from your teacher.

Wednesday night class is taught by an awesome man named Mark. He owns five studios, been teaching seven or eight years, really nice, really positive. He had an interesting start to teaching yoga. His wife was running a Bikram studio and then simply could not go in and teach. I gather she was physically unable. She had a great clientele, big packed classes, and she didn't want the classes to just be canceled. She begged Mark to go in and teach a class for her—the rest is history.

There I am, the uckiest posture por moi, Hands to Feet, knees locked out, hamstrings shrieking. Suddenly, there's my lunch, traveling back up from my stomach, into my throat. I've had the urge to ack before in this posture, but not like this.

The nausea dies down.

I'm in posture #3, Awkward and, blam!, a flash of the violence hits my eyelids. I feel teary and I'm totally regretting not being by Matmate Emily. She'd know what to do.

I let some of the tears out in posture #4, Eagle. I feel like a fool. Most everyone cries at Camel and here I am, crying at the entirely wrong place.

The green-around-the-gills ackiness returns with a vengeance at posture #8, Standing Separate Leg Stretching. Suddenly, I'm weeping. I crave leaving. I'd give up all the water in the world to abscond, bolt, escape, flee, go AWOL, hightail it, skedaddle, vamoose.

Morality Monkey whips out pompoms and reminds me that I'm just the type of gal who sticks things out. I've set the goal of not leaving, and at the halfway point, it would be just plain silly to give it up now.

I tell myself, I won't, I cannot, I will not run screaming from the room. But maybe I should leave. Maybe this is part of growing older and wiser, running from the room; maybe there's no shame in that, it isn't like the door is locked, the door is open just like it was that night in the band hall . . .

. . . and then . . . blam . . .

Like a flash of lightning, I'm back in the room, and I'm remembering the whole thing, the branding, the horse blood, how I got into that room in the first place. Usually my memories of that night are from the floor that I laid on. Seeing the feet and the beer cans and the peanut shells. And later on, in the pre-dawn hours, the grooved rubber mat that I crawled on to leave, and how happy I was that there were grooves as they made me feel like I had regained traction.

This time, though, I'm viewing Kaboom from up above, on the ceiling, looking down. The Kaboom room was the band director's office. And as I tour the memory from above, I see now that the door to the office was open. Wide open.

Oh my god, the door was open and people are milling about the governor and my body is being smashed up against a wall and people see this through the open door and they walk by and look in and everyone is nonchalant and oh god the door was open. Hoards of people walked by and not a single person stopped to help me. No one even stopped and looked concerned or alarmed.

The horror of the scene is unfathomable, bottomless. I've spent my time on the therapist's couch and I do not blame myself any more for what happened. I'm glad I got out with my virginity intact and I'm so thrilled that I do not have a giant branding iron band logo on my rump.

But I think I've always remembered Kaboom night as me against a few evil, drunk cretins. Probably six or eight seniors were in charge of my atonement. So, over time, you can say to yourself, well, that's okay, birds of feather flock together, they didn't hurt your spirit, you can write it off that way.

But the governor standing there, whiskey in hand, ice cubes tinkling in the glass, talking about reelection? And hundreds of people seeing and hearing my personal little torture session with the door open and no one did a thing?

It feels as though I've never cried over this night. I can't even cry with silent dignity. I'm wailing. Here I am, not even at the middle of the class, I'm at posture #9, Triangle, and I cannot contain my overwhelming sense of sadness. I'm sobbing, I have slimy snot running out of my nose, I'm hiccuping, I'm mewling like a 10-day-old kitten who has lost her litter mates.

Plus which, I decided to try the right side of the room and so I'm not near any familiar faces, Matmate Emily is nowhere in sight and she'd know what to do, she's had her share of crying. How can I possibly be so well-attuned to feel love from some freckled ballet dancer and yet have been so out of whack to assume that drunk tuba players would do right by me?

And, ohmygosh, I'm mortified, I feel self-conscious in this new right-side neighborhood, I feel like a reverse fair weather friend. Like I'm cheery and funny on the left side of the room and then all my dreck comes out amongst unsuspecting strangers.

Everyone in the front line starts whispering.

"Doing great."

"Let it go."

"Awesome, you are awesome."

In a way, their unwavering support actually makes the tear spigot go at full blast. We get to halfway, posture #13, Dead Body—our rest between the just-completed standing series and the upcoming floor series. I'm starting to pull my act together and muffle the vocal mewls when the girl next to me touches my hand.

At first, I think, damnit!, what is it with these people invading my mat space? And then I turn to look at her, you know, shoot her one of those "hey!" looks—and she finds my hand and grabs it and squeezes it and then, whatever torrent of tears is now a tsunami.

Has that door-open showing of violence colored me so much that every time someone touches my hand, I think I'm being invaded? I'll bet dollars to (gluten-free) donuts that Darkhaired Dana was trying to be nice and give me an encouraging pat on the hand but I assumed the worst.

The horror of the violence hits me on so many levels that I'm choking now, there are so many tears and wails that need to come out that they are bottled up in the base of my throat.

Evil cretins took my dewy-eyed innocence and destroyed it. The ribs healed and the knees had surgery—but mentally, I'm battered. Even worse, I think, are the ones that stood in the doorway and did nothing. At least the ones that were beating me were being open about their feelings. How awful for me to have had that happen and now, 23 years later, it is ripping my pulpy heart tissue.

I did every single posture, bawling. The teacher, Mark, told some great jokes, so that was nice, to laugh amidst the phlegm.

My hand-squeezing neighbor, a tan and pretty girl named Erica, offered up her half-frozen water bottle. I say no thrice and she says, "You need it, take it." And I wail that much louder at her unexpected kindness. I haven't talked with her that much—though one time we talked about how she was offended at some of Bikram's comments about Jesus. Looking back on it, I chastise myself; I don't think I showed her the compassion she's now showing me.

I love the coolness of the water and I feel the symbolism of it—she's strong enough to go without water and I'm partaking of her strength.

Once I lay down for Final Savasana, I let go and wail.

Suddenly, I have a strong craving for Shannon. I felt that only Shannon would mend the tear.

How very odd of me, though. Shannon and I have spoken maybe three times. She's been through a divorce, and she has heavy hair and a fast metabolism and two kids. That's about the extent of our interaction. I cried at the creepiness of it all, I cried at being embarrassed at wanting her, I cried because I didn't even know her well enough to even know where she usually puts her mat in the room.

I felt a hand on me and I opened my eyes and there was Shannon.

I howled now, as I understand the power of the universe. I was desperate for her and she came.

Someone put a towel over me, a towel still toasty from fluffing in the dryer. Someone else rubbed my feet. Someone else did accupressure on my hands.

And Shannon put her hand right on my rib cage, where I felt all the uckiness of it—anger, panic, fear, loathing. She said, "Let it out," and at first, I said I couldn't, I had already disrupted so much of class.

Shannon smiled and reminded me—she had her own crying class about a week ago. I remember—she shrieked so loudly, you would have thought she was watching someone being set on fire over and over again. And then she napped in the back of someone's station wagon and then her face looked 10 years younger.

Somehow, her hands were pressing right on top of the ucky feeling in my ribs and then the ucky rib feeling slowly went out of me, like a gray wisp of smoke leaving an extinguished candle.

Interestingly, G.I. Jim came over and asked if I was okay—did I need anything? I felt like a fool, but I had to ask, "Did you play trombone in a marching band 23 years ago?"

He shocked me—he smiled so warmly and so compassionately, I cried at my own stupidity for judging him by his crispy exterior. G.I. Jim shook his head and said no. Nice pink underbelly to that man.

Shannon asked him to leave and Adi (pronounced ahDEE, like the beginning of the word Adidas)—a yummy funny exotic Israel-heritage girl who reminds me of Julianne Marguiles—she held my hand and told me to squeeze as hard as I could. I felt so much love and I felt so safe, in my little cocoon and I felt so amazingly blessed to have had my life path end up right here, in a hot room, swaddled in towels, drinking Erica's water—I could not be more blessed.

I knew, down to my bone marrow, that if I had to do it all over again—I wouldn't change a thing. Band hazing was a very small price to pay for infinite, global love and compassion.

THURSDAY 5 MAY

# of days in yoga boot camp: 25

Emmy taught the morning class. Craig had given us a mini-tongue lashing about the evils of leaving class—Emmy had reported on the rush-hour style traffic pouring out of the doors during her Tuesday class. He also stressed that since Emmy teaches Bikram, for the love of god, show the woman the utmost respect.

Then, same thing as yesterday, damnit. Forehead to feet, vomit inching up my trachea. Damnit. Then every posture, the desire to ack is hitting a crescendo and when I swan dive over in posture #8, Standing Separate Leg Stretching—yup—I gotta go. This is more than a bit of ack in my throat.

Horror! Everyone's feet are touching, so I'm doing this odd jumping through the maze dance, trying to get O-U-T out. I end up bumping straight into Emmy and she glowers at me in a way that frightened me almost more than any brand-wielding drunk and I briefly consider going back to my mat to ack there. I consider saying, "Hi, I'm sorry, I really am sick and it is the fourth day of the fourth week and I've never left class, never ever but I've got to go." But if I open my mouth, I know that I will ack directly on Emmy, our future War Stoppage Minister.

Awful violent retching for over a half an hour. I actually craved going back into class—just to be warm and stretch things the other way. Completed the class without too much problem, though I did feel like a sour wrung out washcloth.

I am lucky to get teacher Mark (last night's teacher) for posture clinic and I bang out Balancing Stick with nary an extra word. Well, I caught myself adding two words and then stopped and went on verbatim. Mark said simply, "wow." Asked me what I thought, I said I was a little disappointed in myself, adding the words in and he said, "Just step away from the microphone. Wow."

Interesting—Bikram taught class tonight. I'm feeling awfully weak and praying he doesn't pick on me. And for the first time ever, Miss Pink is left to her own devices.

Although, he did do a hands-on correction, though. In posture #2, Half Moon, he's talking and he takes his fingers and just bends my body so that I'm finally in a half moon shape. I usually look like a crooked chopstick, straight with a little two-inch bend at the top. Suddenly, my body really is crescent-shaped. I look up at him and he smiles down at me and I am in awe of his infinite compassion.

ARDHA CHANDRASANA
HALF MOON

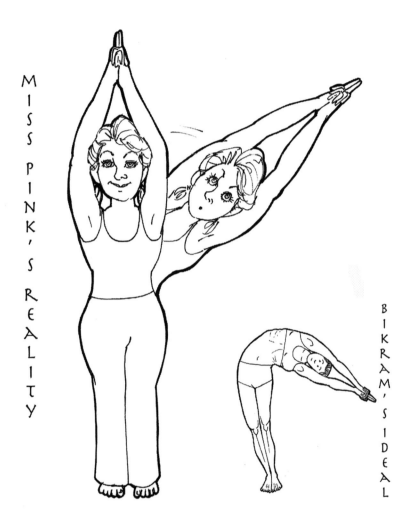

MISS PINK'S REALITY

BIKRAM'S IDEAL

FRIDAY 6 MAY

# of days in yoga boot camp: 26

I think I have miscalculated. I had nine weeks in my head but I was counting again today and I think it is actually 10 weeks, which means we are not halfway.

I managed to grow four quite robust and obnoxious pimples over night.

I guess I'm detoxing, though, so bring it on!

Friday class was taught by Lisa from San Antonio. She's my new hero. She was just an amazing blast of perk and energy and discipline—no room leaving, no wiping hands, no yawning. She had us yell yeehaw during sit-ups and barely said a word of Dialogue verbatim but she just made you want to push harder.

All of the sudden, my Camel is wildly fun. Those intense feelings of panic and anger are gone from my rib cage and I keep looking back and pushing forward and I can see the mat behind me. Wheee!

Physically I'm better but mentally I'm slightly panicked about the Dialogue. My next bit is Standing Separate Leg Stretching and I'd been so obsessed with doing Balancing Stick verbatim—well, I haven't given it much work and what with the crying and acking and pimpling, I've been otherwise engaged. It is my turn to go and I've got G.I. Jim holding the clipboard looking quite unbending. Egads. Breathe. I muster up the courage to stand in front of him—and it is time to go, class dismissed, we have a guest lecture. Hooooray!

G.I. Jim teaches the evening class and he's actually quite good and quite funny. I don't know why, but I sort of expected his decades in the Army to dictate his teaching style. A pleasant surprise, for sure. And then—he lets us go home. Praise be! No monkey lips lecture until midnight.

On our way home, roommate Yok says, "Oh no, you blues eye." What? "Eyes blue." No, hazel. It is the first time we've had a language barrier issue and I find myself feeling quite irritated. I look in the mirror—and I've got a large cluster of broken blood vessels in my right eye.

(Yok was trying to say eye bruise.)

Lovely.

Later that night, standing in front of the mirror, tilting my head in funny ways to try and see the corner of my eye, I feel a tickling sensation, like a spider crawling in my ear. I look over and see coarse kasha-sized nubs of wax flinging themselves out of my ear, as though there's a little chain gang of gremlins in there, tossing out balls of wax.

Funny—the Dialogue often says that the yogi should feel the posture "bones to skin, inside out"—and how! is that ringing true. Short of the toenails shooting off the ends of my feet, I'm not sure what's left.

This healing business is messy stuff indeed.

MONDAY 9 MAY

# of days in yoga boot camp: 29

Decided to try this napping thing. Both Audrey (another Sweatbox teacher) and Saiko stressed to me before I left that the best sleep in the world would be after the class in the morning. I've been dubious about what kind of rest anyone could possibly achieve laying on a smelly sweat-soaked studio floor.

Nonetheless, the fatigue has returned. So I pull my dry towel over me and promptly fall into a deep deep sleep—wake up over an hour later, at 12:15, to the sound of my fellow trainees setting their chairs up for our lecture.

One of Bikram's legal advisers, a nice man named John taught the morning class.

Then, John gave the afternoon lecture on intellectual property and really thoroughly explained the ongoing copyright issue that Bikram has been trying to untangle.

The press has done a great job of confusing the issue; they've made it sound like Bikram is trying to copyright every single yoga posture ever invented since the dawn of time. And they also make it sound like Mr.IOwn85Bentleys is putting the little guy out of business just for the love of money.

Nothing could be farther from the truth.

I was surprised to learn that Bikram has never charged any studio franchise fees—that changes everything in my mind.

Turns out that the origin of the dispute started a while ago, when some teachers decided to change the order of the postures and add a little music to jazz things up. However, they were still calling it Bikram Yoga.

Bikram caught wind of their shenanigans and wrote them a letter, asking that they stop messing with his system. Or, if they were intent on messing with his system, to please stop calling it Bikram Yoga.

The system-messer-uppers got peevish and said they had a right to do as they pleased.

Hatfield McCoy, the prequel.

Lawyer John explained it this way: no one owns a copyright to a piano's 88 keys. Those are public domain and free for anyone to use as they see fit.

However, once you put the notes in a certain order and make a song from the public-domain keys, then you own that pattern, that song. Even the lady who wrote "Happy Birthday" gets royalties for every time the song gets sung.

All Bikram wanted at the outset was to protect his name and his invention. He put 26 Hatha Yoga postures in a specific order and wrote specific words and devised specific heat. The copyright office awarded him a comprehensive copyright. That is, the words + the heat + the order of the postures is owned by Bikram. Change any one element, and it is no longer a Bikram class.

I'm so glad this was all explained. And I think it is important for us to be able to explain this to curious students. I remember my second or third class, I asked the teacher about the lawsuit and all she said was something vague like, "People always are jealous of success."

Bikram taught the evening class, tortured me in Awkward. First I sit down deep enough. I figure that will make him happy.

With a Grinch-ish kind of sly smile he says, "Good. Now heels up Miss Pink. Heels up, heels up, hello, what do you wait for, heels up damnit!"

I get my damn heels up and think, phew, glad that's over.

Bikram starts up again.

"Now Miss Pink, upper body back, not forward, back back back, we all wait for you."

I lean back and I really think something apocalyptic will happen, a vein in my neck will burst or the cellulite will drip from my belly button, but I do it, and I don't fall out, thank gawd and Ganesh.

As we are moving into Eagle pose, Bikram points over at me and snaps his fingers and gets my attention and says, "You did good." I wanted to weep at his unsolicited encouragement.

I did do Dialogue in posture clinic, absolutely verbatim, didn't miss a word, didn't add a word.

I was congratulated for my verbatim success. However, I was informed that I sounded robotic, my precious personality was lost and that's the best part of my teaching, could I please do verbatim with personality? (Apparently not, I wanted to snark.)

The obsession with verbatim is this: Craig told me a few weeks ago that since my presentation skill level was fairly high, he wanted to "set me loose" on to the next level— which is the fun part, playing with the Dialogue a little and making corrections to errant students. However, he wanted me to commit to two weeks of rock-solid verbatim Dialogue, and then he'd let me jump to the head of the class. I do so want to please and honor the flattery that came with his charge—but it suddenly feels like quite a steep hill.

TUESDAY 10 MAY

# of days in yoga boot camp: 27

Did the Dialogue for Triangle Posture today. I think I did blend verbatim and personality—with a few errant words, but I had to add them in! <smirk>

I start out of the gate strongly, feet together, then feet apart then arms down parallel to the floor. Then they bend their knee and you tell them their bent right thigh biceps should look like an upside-down L-as-in-Linda.

I've got their feet apart and their arms down, and oh, horror, I hear myself saying, "Your right thigh biceps should look . . .." Damnit. What comes next? Damn.

Ah yes. Their thigh should look like an upside down letter L. But no sense in telling them that if I haven't gotten them to bend it yet.

My broadcasting training kicks in: never, ever have five seconds of dead air.

So I pause and then said, "Your right thigh biceps should look fabulous in the front mirror."

Raucous laughter and that always makes my cockles warm.

Later on, feeling proud that I was still on the verbatim track, I hear myself saying, "touch your left chin to your left shoulder." Damnit. It is like Tourette's, only less naughty.

The inanity of a left chin and a right chin is hitting and the students are tittering, and my cogs stop spinning because I've just got to prove I can do this verbatim thing, even if that extra word is in there, left chin, can't flunk me cause of that, can they? So I'm trying to keep a straight face, and I say, "your one chin touches your left shoulder . . ." and then I'm blank and there's more laughter and I remember them telling us that if we go blank, to always remember that we are simply telling them what to do, how to do it, and why they are doing it. So to get back on track, I say "touching your chin to your left shoulder because . . ." fuck fuck, the wordsmithy rescue tugboat is not on the horizon . . . so I conclude ". . . touch your chin to your shoulder because you can. And because it looks cool."

Everyone is clapping me on the back, hoorah, I'm funny and the instructor looks at my file and says "Beautiful. Really astonishing. Nice recovery. But—Craig wants verbatim from you."

What the hell do they write in those notebooks anyway?

WEDNESDAY 11 MAY

Recounted my calendar. It really is nine weeks, not 10! Had a rather deep revelation from an unlikely source.

That Asian guy, Egan—the one who told Yok he wasn't Asian, he was Canadian.

Egan annoys me for reasons I know not. He's quite confident and with almost a swagger, an aroma of braggadocio in him. Almost like he's a fancy senior with a car and a Harvard acceptance letter in his back pocket and the rest of us are germy freshmen.

Probably entirely my fault that we didn't get off on the right foot. That first week (which feels like about six months ago), when we were all struggling with Half Moon, he decided he didn't want to say Half Moon in front of Bikram or Craig. Isn't that sassy? So he did nothing, he never went through the rite of passage with the rest of us.

Only reason we find this out is when we finally are done with Half Moon and it is his turn to recite Awkward, he says quite cockily that he'd very much like to say Half Moon as well. Everyone else sort of nods like, okay, sure. I blurt out, "You didn't ever do Half Moon?" And he says no. And I ask why and he says, "The timing didn't feel right to me."

Really now? Can you stand it?

Then about a week later, we are in need of someone to be a student in the mock class for posture clinic and I think it was the week Shannon was crying and napping and there were some injuries and he says, "No thanks, I'm good."

As though he were at a restaurant and the waitress said, "Do you need a refill of your iced tea, Sir?"

I think Leo the Bouncer presses for details and then a gang of us is asking for the why and he says, "I have an injury; my back is a little stiff."

Really now? I've got my kneecap issues and everyone is either swaddled in ice packs or marinating in some version of Ben-Gay. And his back is "a little stiff." Yeesh.

Anyway. Egan keeps adding words and phrases to the Dialogue when he performs in posture clinic. The last time it happened, he said that he felt pretty strongly that Bikram hadn't quite covered the subject he felt he needed to add in.

Can you stand it?

It happened again today. And again, Egan had some kind of sassy reason why the Dialogue coming out of his mouth was better than Bikram's written Dialogue.

A gal from Melbourne, Mili, nudges me with her elbow and rolls her eyes as if to say, "Can you stand it, matey?"

Then it dawns on me. I don't want to be in Egan's club. He's probably a nice man outside of this teacher training boot camp, he's probably some lamb-hugging, celibate, vegetarian leper healer. But right now, the reality is he appears to be arrogant and appears to believe he's smarter than Bikram.

Even if I'm saying goofy things like "Because it looks cool," and even though he's saying things like, "Now before we do the next bit, everyone bend forward from the waist and look down at your feet"—the outcome is still the same.

As I learned a long, long time ago during my stint in Latin America: perception is always much more important than reality.

So I did the Dialogue for Standing Separate Leg Head to Knee tonight, verbatim.

Letitia, a very swell teacher and studio owner from Santa Fe, has proclaimed I am ready for the next level. Hoorah! Victory!!!

I also really value Letitia's opinion. She's very nice and level headed. She sensed that we were a little tired during posture clinic, so she told us a very funny story.

After Letitia came home from her teacher training, she didn't quite have the startup capital together to build a studio, so she taught classes in her house. The room in her house had a heater, mirror and carpeting-and it could accommodate five students. Without the door open, the heat would get pretty intense in the small room.

She had been teaching less than six months and who walks in to her house to take a class, but Jane Fonda. Talk about intimidating! A new teacher, having to teach the Queen of Fitness.

About halfway through the class, Jane Fonda (Fitness Queen!) said to Letitia, "Listen, I'll give you 10 bucks if you just crack the door open a bit."

One of Jane's matmates didn't miss a beat. She quipped, "Jane, offer her 20 dollars; I'll bet she'll open the door then."

In other news, I touched my forehead to my knee today in Standing Head to Knee. I had managed to get low enough to lick my knee with a decent amount of regularity. But this time, the forehead was firmly attached to the kneecap.

I was practicing right next to Matmate Emily (usually she's in the second row and behind me to my left) and I decided that instead of looking at my flawed flanks, I'd do a little mind game.

In my mind, I concocted an elaborate fantasy. Emily and I are roommates in New York City and both are aspiring ballerinas. We are in a dress rehearsal for Swan Lake, with our feather headbands and flouncy giant tulle tutus. And to stretch, before the rehearsal starts, we play around with some Bikram postures and, of course!, my forehead goes on my knee.

Hmm. Wonder if this is the secret to that "mind-body union" that yoga people always gush about.

Craig taught the evening class. I decided to stay next to Emily, directly in front of the podium.

In the middle of the class, the electricity went out. Entire room was dark; no windows in the boot camp torture chamber.

Craig was a god! He didn't miss a beat. I was supping some water, I think it was right after Triangle, and he said, "Everyone, water down, right now, we keep going, we don't need the lights." I not only dropped the bottle on the floor, but I simultaneously spit out the water that was left in my mouth.

Without electricity fueling the giant clock in the back of the room, I imagined it would be a tall order to know where you were in terms of pacing the class. I kept wondering how Craig could cope with such a blind spot. Then realized the stupidity of my query; Craig's been teaching for eons. Must be the same part of my brain that had me informing Steve Forbes that he wasn't nearly as boring as he looks.

THURSDAY 12 MAY

# of days in yoga boot camp: 32

One of my newfound friends is a woman named Julie. She's from Dallas and slightly reminds me of my old psychotic college roommate—but all the good qualities, with the pretension, arson, and shoplifting stripped out.

Dallas Julie (no relation to Strawberry Julie) burst into tears after the evening class. She's been rock-steady, fun to be around, and an easy laugher. We've all been getting increasingly stiff and I can barely get my hands to the floor any more (couldn't even roll my pant cuffs up without bending at the knees)—so we decide to blow off studying at break time and go investigate smoothies.

There's a place across the street rumored to have great freshly-made smoothies. We get there and there's a two-story set of concrete steps and we huff and puff and creak our way up the stairs. I tell Dallas Julie I'm glad we aren't wearing any "Bikram Yoginis in Training" clothing because we look like two newly-sober drug abusers recovering from ingrown toenail surgery.

Smoothie was awesome and hit the spot. And allegedly only 327 calories—such a deal! Pudge Monkey was almost pleased with that food selection.

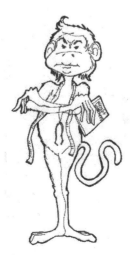

So glad that I didn't have to get up and perform the Dialogue tonight during posture clinic—sugar level high, study level low.

FRIDAY 13 MAY

# of days in yoga boot camp: 33
# of days until I see Prince: 7

Morning class was just wickedly stupid hot, hotter than that other time I said it was hot. Over 40 students left the room and most didn't bother to come back. Rajashree was teaching and you could tell she was peeved. I don't blame her. Made it hard though, as my own mind monkeys wanted to run too.

I had good matmates in my neighborhood though. Kirsten (who is strong enough to live without electricity . . . in Alaska . . . in the winter!) to my right. And Texan Roy to my left and perky Kelly to Roy's left. We held hands during the floor series. At one point, I shouted out "Turtle Power!" and passed on energy down the line, realizing that perky Kelly was probably a toddler during the Ninja Turtles' heyday.

Have I mentioned?

I have the most amazing spouse. We talk every night before bedtime, and it usually goes a little like this:

"Oh my gosh, Hon, it was really hot today."

"Hotter than that other time?"

"Are you talking about that one time at the Sweatbox, when that guy in front of us was sweating little rivers and he splashed us with his sweat?"

"Yes, princess, that is exactly the time I was thinking of. So relative to that class, how hot is Bikram's torture chamber?"

"Well, today, I'd say eight or nine degrees hotter than that day."

"Wow. That's pretty hot. How was posture clinic today?"

"So funny. Mili talked me into going up today . . .."

"Mili from Melbourne?"

"Yes."

"Do you two still have your bet on?"

(Mili bet me that I couldn't say the Dialogue verbatim and, to prove the point, I told her I'd pay her five dollars for each word I added in to the Dialogue. She's quite funny; she said, "Well, are we talking American dollars or Australian dollars?")

And so on. So often I feel like it must be awfully boring for Prince to sit and listen to my nightly not-always-coherent prattle, but here he is, weeks later, remembering little details, like what city Mili is from.

I am so very blessed.

MONDAY 16 MAY

# of days in yoga boot camp: 36

No morning class. I'm not joking. They cancelled the morning class.

It was kind of funny to watch 200 yogis say "huh?" on hearing the news.

Leo the Bouncer made the announcement as we walked in and we were simply unable and/or unwilling to comprehend the concept of no class.

Over a dozen people said be damned, that Leo guy must have it wrong, and laid out mats anyway, in prime mat real estate, ready to capitalize on misinformation.

The class was cancelled to make room for a lecture from a doctor about high blood pressure and the evils of too much sodium in our diet. I felt quite hungry and I snacked on salted almonds.

It gets better. First, we don't have to do sweaty yoga at 9:30 A.M. And then! around 11:00 A.M., miracle of extra miracles, they told us there was nothing on our schedule until after 1:00. P.M.

Yippee! Two extra hours. I studied Dialogue, though I felt slightly ahead of the game, since I put in six hours of studying on Sunday.

The evening class's heat felt like punishment for our idyllic morning of leisure.

One perky Australian gal, Rowena, had her crying breakthrough—and at one point, let out a piercing shriek. Suddenly two shrieks then three and then like an odd Hitchockian amusement park ride, 200 yogis screamed with Rowena. A few folks broke out into gay laughter and then some solemn twits shushed the laughers and then some self-righteous folks shushed the shushers.

In my own little world, I struggled with actually feeling cold and shivery during class.

Today was my big day to switch to Gatorade.

I had done electrolyte water and powders until I realized that was the cause of my heinous gas the first two weeks.

Bikram's wife Rajashree said pishposh on our fascination with electrolyte packets. She believes that all yogis really need is salt, sugar, and lemon in water; maybe experiment with adding ginger for tummy issues and mango for flavor.

Yok and I both switched to Rajashree's recipe, which quickly evolved into an elaborate water-preparation ritual each night.

The semi-alarming news is that a trip to the scales showed an increase of about 12+ pounds on my newly-limber frame. Damn. Tried hard to not obsess about it—but it niggled.

I've been going to a chiropractor on Saturdays after class and turns out he's also a nutritionist. He scolded me for neglecting my electrolytes, said he could feel damage in my C12 muscles (and was even able to feel that I had been bending more deeply in the side-to-side Half Moon posture)—I whined about the weight concerns—but he stressed the importance of going to Gatorade.

I didn't know that Gatorade was invented at University of Florida. The football team needed something more than water to stay perky for bursts of energy performed in extreme heat and humidity.

Chiropractor said that postures in a sweltering Bikram studio would surely qualify for extreme heat and humidity.

I tell him I'm a little freaked about gaining weight with the added calories from Gatorade. I'm shocked by his reply.

He said, "Well, I don't know of a delicate way to put this. As much as you have gained, what's a couple more pounds to protect your muscle fibers?"

He had a point. Though I still felt pretty peevish at his bluntness about my weight gain, which really is all about water retention and the fact that I do have big bones.

I decided if I was going to ditch water-and-mangos, I'd also shake up my mat routine and try out a new neighborhood. I went back to the fourth row, I couldn't see myself in the mirror, all the way over by the doors to the parking lot. Rumor has it, the door mat spots are cooler than anywhere else in the studio.

Well. I was surrounded by fidgety idiots. One woman had a comb and combed her hair, one gal talked and one gal flopped about on her mat and one gal decided to only do every other posture. I honestly felt like I had stepped into another planet.

TUESDAY 17 MAY

# of days in yoga boot camp: 37

Really struggled with the Cobra Pose/spine strengthening series. Felt panicky and hot hot hot and cold and teeth chattered. Not sure what to do with that.

Did Dialogue today with the teacher messing with me—did very well. He followed me around and talked and told me which way to walk, etc. and I hung in there, never strayed from the Dialogue.

Yok's hubby here for another week. He's nice. But I swear to god, he's a Nordic clone of the Prior Husband. Similar traits and ticks and mannerisms—and an inability to take out the garbage.

WEDNESDAY 18 MAY

# of days in yoga boot camp: 38

Such a tough day.

Interestingly, just last week, I had this slight spat with this girl about leaving the room. She said it was her right to leave if she felt hot and I said we needed to stay no matter what. And then she starts saying, well, what if you vomit and I say that's okay and then she says what if you feel dizzy and I say, well, probably not and then she asks who died and made me the rule maker and I want to explain that I always end up the rule maker. I didn't really mean to argue with her, but I felt the need to play devil's advocate.

Anyway, so there I am, in new turf, far away from Melbourne Mili and Strawberry Julie (though Dallas Julie is close by).

For whatever reason, my period decided that 9:55 A.M. on a Wednesday would be a great day to start, catching me very much off guard. First off, it is 11 days late.

(Rajashree even joked, "With the ladies, the periods are all wrong. Either too much or none at all.")

Secondly, it is usually very predictable. The day before, my throat hurts like I'm coming down with a cold and then I feel snipey and then I dive headlong into chocolate and then around 3:00 P.M., it arrives and stays for a tame three days. But not this time.

There I am, in a new 'hood, directly behind TheGalWhoLikedtoLeave. I look down, of course! I have my white yoga mat today, and I see bits of blood and, for a while, I assume that it is the damn feet bleeding again.

The penny-sized blood spots start to merge and by about 10:00 A.M., the blood pool is about the size of a shoebox.

By 10:30, right around the time we move to the floor series, I can stand it no longer. I get up to leave and I see TheGalWhoLikedtoLeave eye me and I swear to god, she felt morally victorious.

Return to class and about 10 minutes later, I'm dripping pink sweat again. Damnit damn damn damn. I can't imagine leaving twice, I just can't. Then, as I was completing a sit-up, I realized with a bit of horror that I was flinging pinkish sweat on my matmates. Eww.

I laid out until the end, did the breathing, and left immediately, with my half-red/half-white yoga mat doing all the talking for me.

I'm embarrassed and horrified and just generally creeped out by the whole experience. Sheepishly, I take everything to the ladies who wash our towels. I have a 20-dollar bill in my hand and I give her the whole bloody mess and she doesn't even blink.

She pauses, looks at me and says, "You okay?"

And I sort of shrug and apologize and offer her the 20 dollars and she laughs and says no, no, its what we do, we wash.

I realized as I showered that I've become a bona fide first row elitist, a mirror-gazing snob. I know Craig has encouraged us to explore new neighborhoods, but why in god's name should I suffer through hyperactive, fidgety, mat-moving energy-suckers? I see no reason.

That, and I'll admit, again, like with the crying, I feel a bit ashamed to have mucked up that neighborhood with my period.

For the first time ever, I'm out of the room before anyone else. I'd dumped my bits with the amazing laundry ladies and am strolling outside and who is standing there in the parking lot?

Sue Peahl! My comedy coach from New York. How awesome. And—how perfectly orchestrated by the universe. We had played email-tag a few weeks ago, trying to pick a time to get together. She moved to L.A. years ago and she's just one of those kindred soul people. She does a lot of neuro-linguistic programming and kindly spent a few hours on the phone with me last fall, helping me reprogram my words and get in touch with my heart's desire.

What an amazing coincidence. The one day I'm not napping, the one day my body demands I leave is the same day Sue shows up.

Also funny to look at the Bikram world from an outsider's eyes. The lined-up purple mats and the taking off of the shoes. The clothing strung out to dry on the wall adds to the imprisoned cult je ne sais qua.

We go out to the garage, I'm telling her about Strawberry Julie (who is nowhere to be found) and Matmate Emily and the heaven called Garage and I see, to her, it is a smelly foul place, littered with unwashed clothing and glassy eyed yoga zealots.

I hated that the visit was so short—haven't seen her in ages. Actually, the last time I saw her, I had started to file for divorce. Sue's still wise, wonderful, Tinkerbell-ish Sue. Wicked funny and profound and lovely and confident and I adore her.

***

Later in the afternoon, Craig mentioned that the smaller room where the advanced students practice—a room typically cooler than the giant room—that the thermometer had flirted with 140 degrees. Only then did they realize that the roof vent was closed—no fresh air could come in -- so that explains the wicked heat.

The evening class was so bad, I did seriously think okay, maybe I go home now. I'm so hot that my teeth chatter, which just can't be a good thing.

I'll just leave. Be damned if I'll be a chronic room-leaver, I'll just go home.

I mean, it would be embarrassing and all, and then it would sound like this:

"Say, didn't you go yoga boot camp?"

"Um, yeah, but I left early."

"Why'd you leave—if you don't mind me asking?"

"Well, you know. It was. Um. Too hot. Even hotter than that one day when that guy splashed sweat everywhere. Stupid hot, you know?"

And then they'd look upon me with pity. And to fumble a bit and tie up the conversation, then they'd quip:

"Oh, okay. I guess, ha ha ha, if you can't stand the heat, leave the kitchen, right?"

And then I'd hear that the rest of my bleeping life. So, to avoid hearing the heat cliché through the dawn of time, I stuck out this evening's class.

Frankie e-mails to say that teeth chattering is a sign of heat stroke. I feel oddly better knowing that, in a twisted, see?-I'm-not-a-weenie kind of way. She also feels very firmly that I need to just leave the room the next time it happens. Dunno. I feel like I used up my emergency room-leaving chits. I must return to my old pledge: I will leave only by stretcher.

THURSDAY 19 MAY

# of days in yoga boot camp: 39

Just a generically great day.

After the morning class, I napped for nearly an hour. There are a good two dozen of us regular nappers; it is nice to know I'm not alone.

I've done well with memorizing the Dialogue and today managed to actually correct students as well. I'll admit, I didn't think I'd get to that point. The gal behind the clipboard had this critique of my performance today: "You will kill them, they will have to crawl out of your studio on their hands and knees." I wish I could put that sentence into a little piece of amber and carry it around with me, maybe wear it around my neck.

Evening class ends on time, right around 6:30. I'm sleepy and I try to fight it and I remember how Prince always reminds me that my body wouldn't ask for it if it didn't need the rest.

(I wonder, though, does that rule apply to chocolate-covered almonds? That my body wouldn't put in the request if it didn't really need the almonds?)

Anyhoo, good golly, I wake up at 7:45. Feeling quite perky but also really hungry. And a bit worried. I'm not sure how I'll shower and snark in dinner and get back in time for our 8:00 lecture. Craig announces that we don't have to be back until 8:30. Yippee! Time to skip across the street and get a smoothie. It is a good smoothie, orange and pineapple with a misting of coconut and life is good, really really good.

Get home in time to browse through email. Bad news. Damnit, damnit, damnit.

Good friend of mine, Barbara is back doing a second round with cancer.

She's already had a hell of a first round with breast cancer. She was such a formidable fighter, you'd think that the cancer cell union would have her put her name on their bulletin board:

MISS PINK

Warning: Do not approach this woman. She appears earthly and vulnerable but, in fact, is armed and quite lethal.

Barbara was eight months pregnant with child number three when she was diagnosed with nonlump inflammatory breast cancer. Who knew cancer could be nonlumpy? That's more creepy than any Stephen King novel. She and husband Dennis had just moved back to the Midwest after a decade in New York.

In fact, their first date was a comedy class—Dennis was in my improvisational comedy class and he brought Barbara along one Thursday night.

Anyhoo, her midwife noticed that the breast was a little stiff. And then labor was induced and chemo and bottle-feeding and awfully bleak statistics. Dennis started an online support group for her and we emailed her well wishes and thoughts and prayers and imagery and then, two blinks, and she's cancer free.

Right next to Jack (a friend of mine who survived 9/11 and whose survival appeared to me in a dream), Barbara's odyssey made me believe again. Believe, in the big capital-B sense. Believing down to my socks in the universe and god(s) and faith and angels and kindness. I believed, nay, I knew that the online support group was the 4000-pound giant blocking tackle as Barbara made her way down the field and spiked the ball and danced her silly knee wubbling dance and declared defeat over all things carcinogenic.

So then. Damn, damn, damndamndamn damnit damn. She's back into the ring with cancer again. They've found four spots that are signs of cancer and I'm just mad. I sort of felt like once I jumped on the Believe wagon, then the outcome would always be cheery. Isn't once enough? She's already managed to swim away from the Titanic of cancer—isn't that enough for one lifetime?

I do know that when they make her Lifetime Television For Women movie, only Meryl Streep or Jeanne Tripplehorn could capture Barbara's big brown Bambi eyes and Wile E. Coyote persistence.

Plus which! She's now working at the hospital where she was treated—they've put her in charge of a complementary care program, her work has just started, it simply cannot be her time to go. Not yet, damnit.

I'm so angry, I want desperately to go and punch something.

FRIDAY 20 MAY

# of days in yoga boot camp: 40

Woke up feeling still mad and a little less Believe-ish and embarrassed, a little, that I'm this twisted and peevish and this mad about Barbara's cancer.

Funny way to start my 41st year, for sure.

Not only is my birthday during yoga boot camp, but it falls on a Friday. Bikram's wife Rajashree teaches on Friday mornings and loves singing to birthday people at the end of class.

I decide to dedicate my class to Barbara. I will think only of her, I will imagine she's sitting beside my mat as I struggle and bend and morph. With her there by my side, I will not succumb to self-doubt, I have no room for that kind of idle monkey chatter now, no, no, I've got to show Barbara that anything is possible. If my foot can come up over my head in Standing Bow, then, for the love of god, she will vanquish cancer again.

Each posture feels like utter perfection, even postures that are easy for me. In Fixed Firm, even, I can really feel my rib cage arching up, and by the end of class, I believe my own promise. I feel like I'm back into the comfy arms of the Believer's club.

After class, Rajashree had my 200 new friends sing Happy Birthday to me. I fight back the tears and sway and enjoy every note of the song.

Rajashree suggested the class dedicate their final breathing to the birthday yogis. I decided I didn't need the energy and the breath—Barbara does. I closed my eyes and imagined the gale-force energy of all that breathing entering me from behind and then me taking that energy and narrowing it to a laser beam and focusing that beam of love and integrity and life-force right onto Barbara's left hip. With my eyes closed, I see four spots, almost like three-dimensional polka dots. I feel like my breath is a pointed blast of air and energy, like a laser beam. I sweep my air laser beam over the four dots, polishing them to sand bits and then the power of the breath blows the sand bits to kingdom come. When I'm done, one dot has just vanished and the other three are a lot smaller.

***

The entire day was a blast! Everyone hugged me and wished me well all day long—even people I hadn't really met yet or socialized with came up and said hi.

(Note to self: do not pout next year when 200 people don't sing to you.)

Prince was due in Friday night, 11:00 P.M. Went to dinner with Dallas Julie. Came home to a message that he had missed his flight and would be due in 12 hours later. I'm relieved, quite frankly. I've hit a wall, fatigue-wise, and even napping hasn't made a dent in it. During dinner, all I could think about was the joy of going home with a full tummy and collapsing into bed.

In other good news—I did get on the scales Friday and I was down seven pounds. That's pretty cool. Gator Power!

Saturday morning—I'm UP nine pounds. Then down five pounds after class. I've spent so much of my life chasing the number, the magic weight number—and attaching my mood and my feelings to each number. I mean, everyone does this. At 138 pounds, I'm giving Christy Brinkley a run for her money and life is gay and delicious. At 144 pounds, I'm mostly happy but my skin is less shiny. At 155 pounds, I wonder why someone hasn't taken me out and shot me, the way you do a horse with an irreparable broken leg.

But now, with nine-pound swings in one day, who can keep up?

MONDAY 23 MAY

# of days in yoga boot camp: 43

Morning class was taught by this great woman named Carolyn. Another old-timer Bikram teacher, another ageless stunning doyen.

First time in ages that I felt like a student again. No Miss Pink pressure, no boot camp expectations. Just focused on doing the posture right. I actually felt brave enough to ask for help with the Standing Bow Pulling Pose – I've felt so stymied.

I finally get my foot back over my head—but then I seem to stall out at that point. The teacher told us to raise our hands if we wanted help—she came by and held my stretching (nonankle-grasping) wrist and said, "now kick kick kick."

I said, "I think I'm crooked."

She said, "Who cares? Just kick, for the love of god. Kick!"

Oh my, the feeling of the power of my kick, of my shoulders really being pulled apart.

Wow.

Craig started tonight's lecture with, "Well, congratulations on surviving anger week."

Immediately, I was filled with red-hot molten lava anger. How could he have not told us? Why is he so cheeky about these things? What an amazing asshole! I could not believe I ever thought he looked like a young Costner. Costner! Pshaw. Right now, he looks like Chucky, that possessed doll with spiky red hair.

DANDAYAMANA DHANURASANA
STANDING BOW PULLING

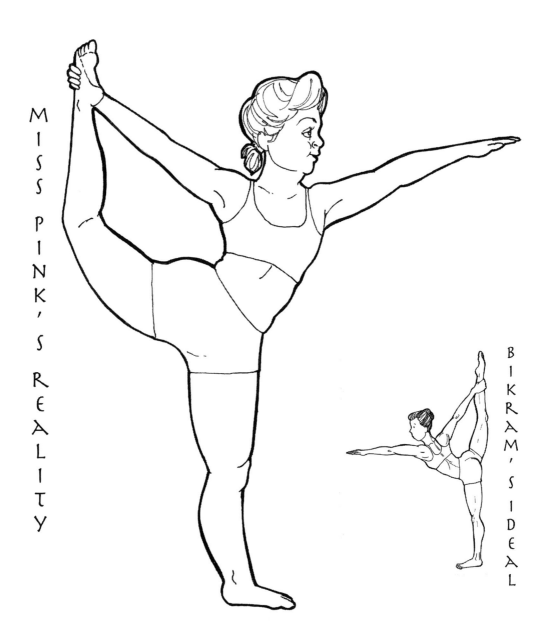

MISS PINK'S REALITY

BIKRAM'S IDEAL

TUESDAY 24 MAY

# of days in yoga boot camp: 44

I'm really enjoying my newfound friendship with Melbourne Mili. She's quite funny and we save seats for each other. She's been great when my confidence has flagged lately.

I had been feeling like quite the rock star with the Dialogue—I had memorized the first nine postures before I arrived. So while the rest of the world was flipping out on weekends and rocking in the corner with an iPod blaring the magical Dialogue words, I went to the chiropractor and napped and watched movies and went to bed early.

Now, however, I've gone over the horizon of my flat world, and I feel a lot less confident in my ability to say the words precisely. I know beyond a shadow of a doubt that I'll be fine teaching it with less-than-exact words.

Mili notices this and tells me I've got to get off my duff. I've got to get in the line to perform the Dialogue, and then do what everyone else does—memorize on-the-fly, sitting in the line, heart pounding, sweating, mouth dry. I do not like Mili's plan at all.

There I am, enjoying my happy little yoga universe and then, like a bucket of ice water dumped on your unsuspecting head in the midst of a nice steamy shower—an odd confrontation.

My upstairs neighbor Denver has really struggled with staying in the room. He leaves pretty much every class and often stays gone. I'll admit, the snarky side of me wonders if they'll graduate him. If he can't stay in the room to take a class, how can he possibly stay put to teach a class?

He's actually a very nice person otherwise. He plays guitar and a perk of him being my neighbor is that he'll stay up later than I do and play his guitar and I adore having that to fall asleep to. I'm Pavlovian about it, really. I hear a couple of chords, and my eyelids droop big and fat and heavy and I wake up refreshed.

(Note to self: buy a CD from Denver before graduation.)

Anyway, Craig announced that we will have a talent show next week. I toyed with the idea of hosting; otherwise, I don't really have any showcase-able skills.

Like an undefeated whack-a-mole, Denver pops his head up and says he will run the talent show. Humph. At first, I'm thinking, well, well, who died and made you king? And then I find my breath and think actually, he'd be a really fun person to play with, comedy-wise.

Yok is tapping her teensy foot, she's always anxious to bolt into our car and get home before everyone else (thereby ensuring maximum sleep time). She's so intent on getting home, I do think she'd happily cut Bikram off in traffic if it meant her getting home before him.

But today, but I figure, screw it, I'm not going to bolt from the studio every single time. I still haven't quite figured out who my Best Friend for Life is going to be (though I am rooting for Mili) and the clock is ticking. Good god, only 18 days until graduation!

Anyway, I said to Mili that I really wanted to be part of the talent show.

Mili tells me to just go over and ask Denver. That if I say nothing, then it will be my spirit that died and made him king. Gosh, she's deep some times.

She's right. I go on up and tell Denver I'd love to help with the hosting.

He looks angry, his brows squinch up and his eyes turn icy and he just says no. He doesn't even stop and ponder, he says, no, no, he's a professional; he does this for a living.

(Hmm. Didn't he say he worked at a sushi restaurant?)

I said that a two-hour gig is long for anyone, and if he needs any help . . .

Before I can finish the sentence, he cuts me off and says he's working with Jude from Australia. That Jude has a lot of energy and enthusiasm and he's looking forward to giving her on-the-job training with this talent show.

And that, quite frankly, he only wanted to work with "true professionals."

I so desperately wanted to say, well, Mr. Guitarboy, I'm not sure but I do think live radio and television slightly counts as professional, as do my years of training in Chicago City Limits, and performing a master class in da big apple would qualify, a teensy bit, for being a professional, and then Mili said I should breathe.

Mili asks, "What about that novel you've shoved into the drawer? Wouldn't it be fun to read that out loud?"

Maybe she has a point. Maybe.

Clearly Yok's 100-yard car-dash has served me well these past few months. Absconding so quickly from the yoga pod has helped me avoid negative interactions.

Gained 10 pounds this morning, lost 7 during class. Biggest one-class drop yet.

WEDNESDAY 25 MAY

# of days in yoga boot camp: 45
# of days until graduation: 17

Mili is awfully wrong about the talent show thing. Why do I allow myself to be so swayed by other people? I read through the signup sheet for the talent show, and I feel like such a nerdling. Everyone else is doing exciting things, like playing instruments and singing and karate and physical things. Reading a novel—yawn! Plus which, I'm just not sure it would play well, either.

I decide I'll rally my fellow comic gals, it'd be way more fun to do a skit with them.

Kay assured me she is a one-woman-act kind of gal. She was quite firm about it.

That leaves Redhead Amy from New York. She's wicked funny and has talked about really struggling with a creativity crisis. Maybe she hasn't really done that much performing yet and this would be a great laboratory for her?

So I sort of dance around that issue, that maybe she should restart her creative juices in a smaller audience and she tilts her chin sideways and then I ask her what exactly she has done performance-wise and then I think her eyes sort of got crossed. I backed off that, clearly I was hitting some kind of sore spot with her. I ask if she's ever taken any kind of comedy classes and she's shaking her head, poor thing, and then I said maybe just a round of the classic improvisational game BippityBippityBop would reignite her confidence. She says something about only working solo and I feel I've alienated her.

Either that, or I just plain smell funny.

(Note to self: investigate new deodorant choices this weekend.)

Funny, two nights ago, during a break, she was talking about pressure from her family and I said she should tell her family to piss off, who are they to judge comedic talent anyway? I sometimes wonder if she's been brought up by a family of dentists or Amish people and all they want for her is to drill rotten teeth or rebuild fallen barns.

Bikram taught today's evening class—he's been in Japan for over two weeks. Very nice to have him back home; I've really missed him.

MISS PINK

I thought perchance Bikram would have forgotten about his Miss Pink plaything. He was silent in Half Moon and stared a lot at me in Awkward and Eagle, still nothing.

Although I sort of felt ignored by him, I realize that it is nice to be in my own little world with my postures, left to my own devices.

I'm at Standing Separate Leg Stretching, and to be honest, I've spent a lot of time feeling mad at this posture. There's this giant emphasis about touching your forehead to the floor—which hasn't happened for me, so I sort of resent the whole endeavor.

Last Saturday, Matmate Emily said, "You are so close to getting your forehead to the floor!" I'm thrilled to hear this, it always feels like the floor is miles from my head. Then all my mat neighbors are jumping in with suggestions and tips and voila!, my forehead touches the floor.

I'm so psyched, and Bikram's been staring at me, I feel like "Check this out, daddy-o! Lookie here! My forehead is finally on your damn floor!" Seriously, if I could have wagged my tail at the man, I would have.

Bikram leans over the edge of the podium. Here we go again, he's the Jungle Book snake. I know, intellectually, that he's at least three feet away. Still, I feel as though his face is next to my ear and his breath warms the hairs on my neck. He hisses, "Ah. Now, with your forehead on the floor, you need to grab your heels Miss Pink."

I was thiissss close to my heels, maybe one inch away. I semi-ignore him, what does the man want from me? Can we not just take a couple of classes and celebrate my forehead victory?

"Grab your heels, grab your heels, Miss Pink, grab your damn heeeeeelsss."

Damnit. My left hip is shrieking, my hamstrings are on fire, I finally get my right hand within a few millimeters of the heel neighborhood, the left hand flies out spastically, knocking over Matmate Emily's water and then my shoulder hurts and he says, "We will all wait until Miss Pink grabs her damn heeeeels."

Bless it! I'm relieved right now that only a handful of people know I'm Miss Pink. I don't even think Mili knows. Special moments like this and I worry I'll be shunned from the whole group, just like that whole first grade porridge standoff.

(I lived in Wales during first grade and second grade. The Welsh people were crazy for putting porridge on top of luscious desserts. Awful gray vomit-looking stuff. So I said "no thank you," which little Welsh girls were not supposed to say. The teacher announced that there would be no midday recess if I didn't eat my porridge. I didn't care, the peer pressure was white hot, but I refused to eat the porridge. For days and weeks on end, the entire school did not have recess, which made me quite the social pariah.)

So there we all are, all 200 yogis, waiting for porridge-averse Miss Pink to grab her damn heels. My hand keeps flying out and then once I got the left hand closer to the left heel, the right hand gave up its battle and flung out and smacked the mirrored podium and he sighed and said the magic "change" word and I'm relieved he saw it was a losing battle.

DANDAYAMANA BIBHAKTAPADA PASCHIMOTTHANASANA
STANDING SEPARATE LEG STRETCHING

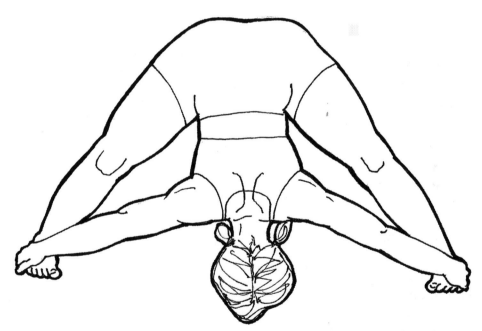

MISS PINK'S (DARN AWESOME) REALITY

Mili saved me a seat for the evening lecture. We were early (or, more likely, the lecture was running late), so we had time to gab. I'm not sure how we wound our way to the topic of self-esteem, but we did. I sighed a war-weary sigh and said, "You know, must be nice to wake up and look in the mirror and feel great. What an amazing way to start off your day, you know?"

She snapped her gum and thought for a few seconds and said, "But it is your mind. You can tell it to do anything you want it to do."

Hmm. Dunno. She's got quite perfect tan legs and a nonround face where you can actually see the jaw line. Maybe things are different in Australia.

Frankie emails and throws down a challenge: no more hopping on and off scales until one month after I come home.

Initially, I think, well, okay, all well and good for you normal-weight Civilian people, but some of us have to monitor these things very carefully. But she's about to be my new boss, so, all right, fine.

THURSDAY 26 MAY

# of days in yoga boot camp: 46
# of days until graduation: 16

Pretty darn stiff and sore from last night's work out—there is a lot of hobbling and creaking and helping each other out of the car. If week #6 was Anger Week, then I dub week #7 StiffAsABoard Week. (And while I'm not weighing myself, I know that I am not light as a feather.)

Sometime during Emmy's marathon morning class, with my forehead on my knee, sweat running into my eyes, I did think to myself, "Eff the yoga. The novelty of this gig has worn off, I really could use a day off."

Bikram taught the evening class. And corrected me—oodles and oodles.

In fact, he corrects one gal and says if she can't figure out how to do the breathing, then to look at me—how amazing is that? I've always worried my first breathing exercise was off somehow, my elbows don't hug my ears like the other yogis.

There we are, back in the sit-on-invisible-chair Awkward Pose, and we begin our little dance. "Sit down Miss Pink, sit down more." Fine, I can do that, I know exactly where he likes it.

"Miss Pink, heels up, lean back more, get your damn heels up, lean back, not forward, lean back lean back. Hello? Do you not hear me? Mooooore back."

So I lean back on his command and then—I'm literally ass over tea kettle, I fall so hard and so unexpectedly that I roll into an uncontrolled summersault, backward, into the second row, nearly knocking over the tallest trainee, a man Bikram has nicknamed LampPost.

Then on to Eagle.

Bikram has repeatedly said, "If you can't wrap your foot, use your damn hands."

So I always look at him like, "What da hell you talking about?" First off, he's squealing at me to interlock my fingers at the beginning of Eagle so that I'll get that all ipsy pipsy twisty pretzel perfect. Then now what? How exactly do I use my hands? Should I uncross them to push my foot? That isn't in the Dialogue, you know, I mean, I hate to be snarky, but it isn't, and I feel silly, I mean, should I keep the arms wrapped around each other?

I'm running through all these questions and he barks out, "How many time I have to tell you Miss Pink, use your damn hands."

I untwisted my pretzelized hands/palms and it worked! I got my foot shoved back and hands/palms re-twisted without too much drama.

(note to self: Bikram brainwashing appears complete. Who in their right mind says handspalms? Let alone thinks it? Hie thee to www.Amazon.com to buy book on cult deprogramming.)

I'm feeling kind of tired in Standing Bow. And defeated. I mean, honestly, I look at Emily and her calf muscle is over her head. I just don't think that's in my future.

"You not kick at all Miss Pink, you just stand there, I can tell these things."

So I kicked and then he got a happy twinkle in his eye and said, "Now you kick harder, good, good. I know you can kick even more."

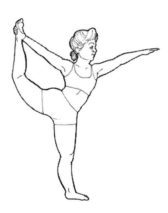

How is it that Bikram sees my abilities and I do not? Maybe he just doesn't understand pear-shaped Lutheran girls. I do know, I'm 100 percent certain that he does not have warring monkeys running about in that head of his.

I decide after class to use the Savasana to tidy up my mind monkeys, bring some sense of order to them. I don't think Bikram is pretending to believe in me. He sees something I do not see and, honestly, something I have never seen.

That, and quite frankly, I'm so tired of them and their monkey shenanigans.

They got into a huge brawl during Standing Bow today, Pudge Monkey and Money Monkey united. Pudge reminded me that calves are so fat, I have to special-order boots. And that it is best left that way, with my calf not over my head. Emily's calf goes over her head because she's thin and has pretty legs. Money Monkey chimed in with moral support; perhaps Bikram hasn't noticed my fat calves yet. Why risk it now? And, more importantly, why risk it and lose the tuition investment?

Shopping Monkey tried to come to my defense, with a list of nearby tanning salons – the spray-on kind – that would make my legs prettier.

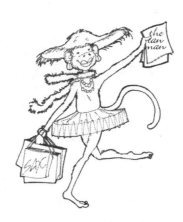

She had a great point, Shopping Monkey. Tan legs always look better than my current Casper the Friendly Ghost white.

Pudge and Money kicked Shopping in the shins. Morality Monkey tried to come to the rescue, but Pudge flattened him with a shockingly strong right hook. With Morality Monkey unconscious, there was no one left to defend my honor.

I closed my eyes and imagined walking up stairs to my brain. Narrow stairs, maybe only 18 inches wide, and well-worn in the center.

At the top of the stairs was a fairly organized place, not too big, not too small. Reminded me of my grandma's attic. Dormer-style slanted roof, lathe-and-plaster walls, smells of sunshine and rain.

I see no monkeys. Odd. I hear some skittering and I notice that the monkeys are hiding behind old suitcases to the right of the door. Morality appears to be still unconscious, lying flat with an ice pack on his head. Pudge, Shopping and Money are huddled together. They have all done their best to disguise themselves. Pudge is wrapped in many, many tape measures. Money has his hands over his eyes. And, of course, Shopping monkey made time to buy an entirely new outfit for her disguise.

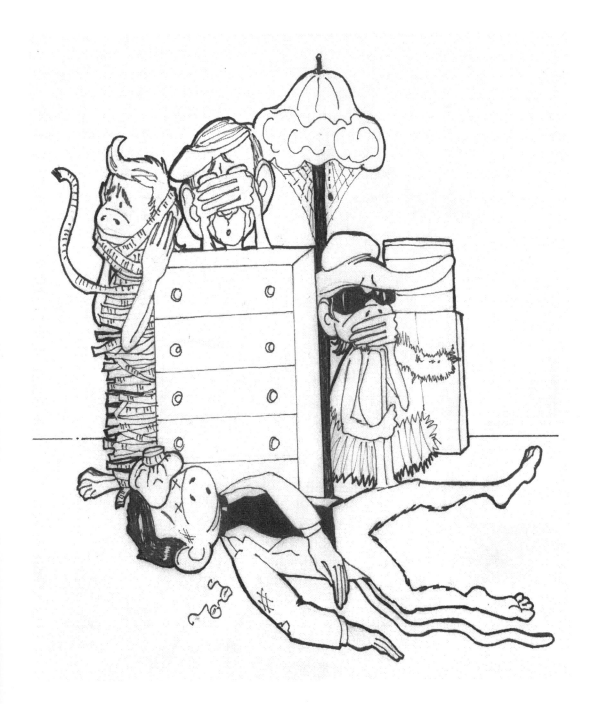

In the center of the room is a dragon, stereotypical forest green dragon, lighter Key lime green underbelly, red forked tongue. Scattered on the floor are Pudge's body fat caliper, Money's calculator, Shopping's hat and a large, serious-looking book I presume to be Morality's.

I approach the dragon and she issues a big plume of standard-issue fire breath. Then nothing, silence.

"Is that all you've got, trick-wise?" I ask.

"Go away. You are retaining water. You should leave now, otherwise your legs will swell and you won't be able to go back down those stairs," she hissed.

"Listen, can we talk about why you are here?"

"Why wouldn't I be here?" she snapped.

"Most sane people don't have mean-spirited dragons in their heads."

"How would you know about sanity?"

"Are you a Jewish dragon?"

"Why do you ask?"

"Because you seem to be answering everything with a question," I clarified.

"So it's not that I'm a dragon, but that I'm a Jewish dragon?" Her pitch was snivelly and I think I sensed panic in her voice.

"It isn't that you are Jewish. It is that you are mean, obnoxious, a bully."

I couldn't quite finish my laundry list of reasons why I don't like dragons of any religious faith, and I hear whimpering. And then the dragon mask falls off. It isn't a dragon at all. No, no, it is a regular human dressed up in a dragon costume. Though, I'm not sure if this helps me at all, in terms of a mental wellness credit report.

I walk over and she lifts her head—and—to my shock and horror—I see my Sunday School teacher from 1969. Cat-eye glasses, beehive hairdo, the whole 60s mod thing.

"What the hell are you doing in disguise in my brain? Shouldn't you be back in Pennsylvania?"

"Watch your language, young lady! Listen, you have always been a troublemaker. It was simply my job, my calling, to keep you on the straight and narrow."

"How in god's name could I have been a trouble maker at age five?"

"Oh, I taught you until you were 11. When I retired . . .."

Her voice trails off and she starts murbling words into her once-perfect starched hanky. She regains her exposure, licks her chubby manicured dragon talons and applies her spit to her beehive, which had become a little more haystacky than hive-ish.

"Don't you remember how you tormented me? With all those questions? Like if Jesus is the king of Jews, shouldn't we switch too? Why does our 'nice creed' say we believe in the catholic apostolic church—do they believe in Lutherans?"

"But aren't those normal children questions?"

"Never you mind."

"Listen, I can't have you in my head any more. You aren't nice at all and . . .."

"If I leave, who will watch over you? You know, last night at dinner, you had an overload of 634 calories. If I'm not there, you'll wind up like your Aunt Katherine."

"Well, no, I won't. She was diabetic. And an alcoholic."

I notice the dragon is fading and shrinking in size.

"And she had gland issues that they didn't have medicine for. Plus which, Katherine was a big baby, 14 pounds, and she was a big child who never got smaller. I'd know by now if I were destined to become a 400-pound drunk."

In the corner, there was nothing left but the shriveled up dragon costume and a pair of cat- eye glasses. I thought I heard hissing; I leaned over and Sunday School teacher warbled, "I can come back at any time!"

I turned around and the tidy attic was well-lit and there was a vanity and a sweet little monkey. Me, I think. Sort of looked like me. She smiled and opened a closet door, brimming with boas and rhinestones and tutus. She donned a tutu and a large brimmed hat, and flopped on the bed, content.

FRIDAY 27 MAY

# of days in yoga boot camp: 47
# of days until graduation: 15

The good news is that with the power of my mind, it was the first morning in ages that I just got out of bed and started my day. No looking in the mirror for extra pounds, no poking at thighs, no sadness that they aren't supermodel thighs—I just upped and brushed and the mind was quiet. Well, not exactly quiet as my inner me was cheering, pom-poms a-rustle. But the nagging dragon was still d-e-a-d.

The bad news is that I had a helluva time actually leaving the bed. Stiff stiff stiff—like the day after my knee surgery stiff. Getting out of the car is slightly comical—though as I was oomphing my way out of Yok's 2-door sports car—the uber-hiking/running gals parked next to me had a hard time dismounting their Jeep.

We get out of class early, which is always such a treat.

Mili and I have plans for the weekend. So very excited—she got tickets to Universal Studios theme park. And not any kind of tickets; VIP passes, which means we get to go to the front of the line. Won't that be awesome?

Come home to best news ever. Barbara's husband Dennis writes to say that there are now only 3 cancer spots. There were 4 and now there are just 3 and they've decided against surgery.

And, most awesomely, he concludes:

"I felt very small against the powerful gift you offered to Barbara. 200 hot and sweaty yogis breathing for Barbara. The only comparison I can make is the first time I saw the ocean. Beyond comprehension that something could be that big, yet there it was."

I sat and wept at the beauty and serendipity of it all. Meeting Dennis and Barbara on their first date. If I hadn't had my own breast scares, I doubt I would have ever gone to the Sweatbox in the first place.

Up until today, I've never really thought my writing skill had any place on this planet.

Suddenly, here, in my rental property in the midst of yoga boot camp, a teary, bleary-eyed email helped a friend in need.

Good stuff. I will put my name on the signup sheet tomorrow for the talent show. Hopefully it isn't too late.

SUNDAY 29 MAY

# of days in yoga boot camp: 49
# of days until graduation: 13

Had such a great day with Mili. We went to Universal Studios and had a blast. It was great to worry less about money—since the tickets were free, we splurged on lots of things. First off, I was more than happy to pony up extra money for extra-close VIP parking. We did a ton of rides—an easy feat once you have a magic bit of paper hanging around your neck that entitles you to go right to the front.

I had a temporary tattoo of dolphins put on my ankle and Mili bought some fun T-shirts for friends back home.

On our way out of the park, we stopped at an oxygen bar. (Only in L.A. do they have "bars" for oxygen.)

The oxygen bar had interesting new age-y toys and books as well. As we were about to leave the oxygen bar (neither one of us wanting to actually pay $17 for oxygen that we already breathe for free, albeit not pina colada scented), I spotted a basket with little round metallic pebbles with words engraved on them, like joy and happiness, etc.

Mili paws through the basket and pulls out three and puts them in front of me.

"You know, you've got so much to offer. And yet, you have always allowed people to steal these from you. Now's the time for you to reclaim them and never let them be taken from you again."

I looked down and the tiles read: Harmony, Growth, Joy.

How did she know that? Gosh that's deep.

MONDAY 30 MAY

# of days in yoga boot camp: 50
# of days until graduation: 12

Woke up feeling a little sun burnt from our fun day. And creaky stiff. My throat's a little sore, too, but I did have Betty's top down most of yesterday.

This morning's class was, simply, no fun. I felt desperate for anything other than yoga.

I started out by trying to shake things up. Put my mat in a new neighborhood, staying on the left side of the room, to avoid the hair combing gal on the right side. Back five rows, and just a few spots over from the big double fire exit doors. Felt sick from all the car exhaust trickling in from La Cienega Boulevard. Several people came over to ask if I was okay—no pink and no front row?

The great news is that Saiko is in town. Somehow, seeing her makes this more real, it pulls thread from my non-yoga-pod life back into my existence, a life that includes a precious Prince and chai tea and yoga on a whim, not on demand.

We plan to take evening class together—I told her about the morning trek to the car exhaust side of the room and she shook her head and said, no, no, you like the front row, that is where you should always be.

My knees were really stiff and I wanted to really put on a good show for Saiko; no sense in putting on my suffering show for a visitor and soon-to-be coworker. I had bought some magic ancient-Chinese-secret pain-remover at Whole Foods. I broke open the bottle. It said, "Use sparingly."

Rubbed about two drops onto my knees, especially in the back, and nothing. Then two more drops, nothing. Then eight drops, nothing. Hmm. Maybe ancient-Chinese-secrets have expiration dates?

I go in the room to put my mat in my spot. Damnit! My favorite front row spot is taken. I move about five spots down and then I feel the flames. A small brush fire has broken out on the backs of my knees, my poor little legs are cherry-tomato red. I have petite prickly tears running down the sides of my face, not emotional tears but the too-much-wasabi kind of spontaneous leaking.

I run to the bathroom and turn on the cold water. And then hot water. And then cold again. I scrub with a washcloth and soap—nothing. Beet, beet red legs. I go into the steam room, and oh no, steam is not the answer to flaming thighs. I go back into the shower and am struggling to get the water right onto the backs of my knees. Then it occurs to me— Balancing Stick! I do a lovely Balancing Stick and the cold water pelts my poor besieged skin. Sometimes this yoga really comes in handy!

TULADANDASANA
BALANCING STICK

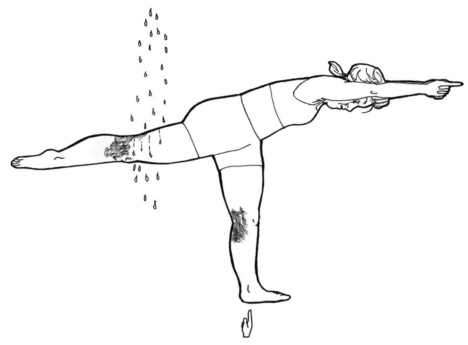

MISS PINK'S REALITY
BIKRAM'S IDEAL

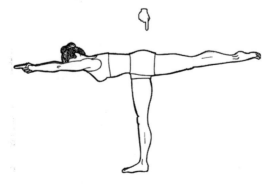

With the fire (mostly) out, my chills during class came earlier today. Usually, I start feeling cold by the floor series. Today, my teeth start chattering by the fourth posture, Eagle.

Bikram gave me zero corrections. And that has me worried. He has a well-honed sixth sense as to how people are feeling; I must be bad off if he's letting me be.

Someone gave Bikram a digital camera right before class and he's like a little kid with a freshly unwrapped Christmas gift. He has us holding postures for minutes on end as he clicks and points and oohs and aahs. I think we were in Balancing Stick for a good two minutes. He gave us a break and we collectively huff and puff. He discovers the shot hasn't quite come out the way he wanted, so we go back for another epic Balancing Stick.

The entire class is about him and camera and getting good shots. The shivering is only getting worse, so for the first time, I laid out. I simply did not have the strength for Cobra. Or Locust. Or Full Locust.

Bikram comes zooming over to our side of the room and stands an inch from my big toes and all I could think was that I'd have no choice, I would have to get up and do the damn Floor Bow so he could get his perfect shot.

He kicks my foot and then I think, oh, crap, now I'm really in for it. I look up and he leans in close and whispers, "Miss Pink! Are you okay?"

I look into his eyes, searching for malice. And all I see is genuine concern and compassion and little puddles of tears plump out my bottom eyelid.

I didn't know what to say, really. I couldn't exactly say, "You know, Boss, actually, I'm quite cold." Good god, he'd have a field day with that.

I made a Mr. Yuck face, complete with protruding tongue, and he smiled and said, "Then you take it easy today Miss Pink. Okay?"

I gave him a thumbs-up and returned to my Savasana.

TUESDAY 31 MAY

# of days in yoga boot camp: 51
# of days until graduation: 11

Cannot believe we are so close to graduation—10 days away! Bikram kept us until way past midnight, talking about marriage and men and women. Didn't pay too much attention. Instead, focused on Dialogue and got two pages memorized as he spoke. Almost feels like my memorization is going more smoothly. I'm still so glad, though, that I got as much Dialogue stuffed into my brain as I did before I arrived.

WEDNESDAY 1 JUNE

# of days in yoga boot camp: 52
# of days until graduation: 10

Rajashree did a great lecture today, starting to touch on modifications and illnesses and things to be on the lookout for. Christelle, a very funny sprightly gal from Ibiza, stood up and asked about getting cold during class. Hoorah! I'm not alone. My ears prick up, I cannot wait to hear the answer, the cure, the way to make it stop.

Rajashree said simply, "Well, that should not be happening." She did talk for some time about all the many different reasons for chills to happen. Low blood sugar, low blood pressure, fatigue. She looked at Christelle (who has about 5 percent body fat) and said, "Well, for you, I'd say it is most likely because you have such low body weight and maybe too much water."

Well, damnit, now I cannot stand up and ask the question again. First of all, I wouldn't want to annoy Rajashree and second of all, I fear the answer. "Well," she'd say, eyeing my little pear-shaped body, "For you, you have so much body fat and you do freeze your water, yes? Then I'd say the frozen water is settling into your body fat and expanding as it melts."

Frankie has been emailing pretty insistently, saying that the chills are serious and I've got to address them. Even if it means asking Bikram or Craig.

I took a big giant inhale and asked Craig.

As I suspected, he immediately found the humor. "Too cold, huh? Poor thing. Shall we turn the heat up then?"

Bah.

He did say it was a great question and he wasn't sure he had the answer. Was I eating okay? Hydrated okay? Healing crisis, perchance? I said I wanted to have a good answer should a future student of mine have a similar issue.

"You know what? Ask Bikram."

Well, that's not bloody likely, not at all. Bikram and I have enough issues as it is, I'm not about to give him something new to torment me with.

The most probable answer came from an Australian flight attendant named Anna. (I gotta tell you, I just love the gang from Australia. They are all so very nice and cheery.)

Anna specializes in really, really long haul flights. She's learned over the years that severe fatigue's #1 symptom is temperature regulation issues. After she gets off a long flight, she's bursting with heat—and by the time she gets home, she's freezing, she cannot get warm. So I'll vote for that right now.

Worked my ass off in class today. For the first time in ages, I felt like I was really breaking through some plateaus in some of my postures. Got my forehead on my knee for over one nanosecond in Head to Knee, kicked like a wild mustang in Standing Bow, forehead thunked to floor when appropriate.

Cold shivers and teeth chattering came in the floor series. I felt as though I could roll over and nap. Then I thought, "Screw it, I won't leave the room, but I'll just do a teensy little baby Cobra pose." Out of nowhere, I started mentally humming the "You deserve a break today" song. Then wondered if it was McDonald's or Burger King that thought I needed a break. And the song is making me really happy and content with my frigid little Cobra. I've found the happy spot, I have, I can hum and sort of phone in the posture and then I hear:

"Miss Pink, what the hell is that? That is not a Cobra. You do nothing. At least use your hands to push up. Look at me Miss Pink, how many times I have to tell you: 99 percent right is 100 percent wrong."

Blah blah blah. Whatever Calcuttaboy. Ninety-nine percent is all I got for you today.

Second set, he says, "Miss Pink, look at me. You have got to use your hands in Cobra, like Dialogue says. Use your goddamn hands Miss Pink."

Oh fuck. He sounds mad. I swear this is a trick. But he hasn't ever seemed angry before and I look over and his black diamond eyes are dark pools of venom.

Well, I've gone this far, I've honestly got to defend my honor.

"But it isn't in the Dialogue."

"What?"

"The Dialogue says 'use 100% spine strength.'"

"So use your damn spine, then Miss Pink."

"Um. Okay. But I do use spine strength."

"That's all you have? Your chin is off the floor maybe one inch Miss Pink."

"Yes boss."

BHUJANGASANA
COBRA

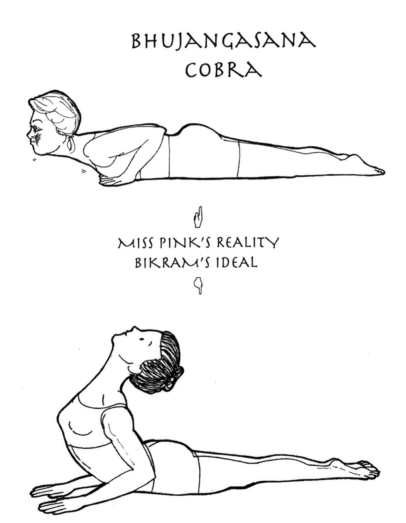

MISS PINK'S REALITY
BIKRAM'S IDEAL

Blahblahblah, I'm not using my "junk body" and onandon, with at least one mention of my "cottage cheese ass."

I want to go home.

THURSDAY 2 JUNE

# of days in yoga boot camp: 53
# of days until graduation: 9

Worked my ass off in the morning class and felt like it barely showed. I'm stiffer than I've ever been in my life and my muscles seem to be intent on hardening more and more.

I was really dreading the evening class. Broke down and got an ice pack. Took an hour to figure out where the ice pack would even go. Left knee, left ankle, left buttock, left nipple (the nipple! that's just plain freaky), right clavicle, right inner knee—all are wounded to varying degrees. The freaky nipple pain takes my breath away and then I see buzzing white spots in the outer edges of my vision.

Decided the ice pack would be best put to use on my right knee. I've avoided the ancient Chinese secret stuff since last week's arson.

The evening class was quite a pleasant surprise. Diane from Boston taught. Up on the podium, she looked a bit mousey and timid, almost like she should have been a librarian.

Diane's yogic journey almost sounds like a fairy tale. In 1985, Diane bought a book by Raquel Welch that details the Bikram yoga sequence. Diane's mom, meanwhile, knew a woman named Madelyn who was teaching Bikram's yoga series in a nearby dance studio.

Over time, Diane started teaching when Madelyn was unable. Diane found out that Bikram was alive and well and offering teacher trainings. She attended Bikram's second teacher training in 1995. There were only 30 people attending and no written Dialogue to obsess over. All the posture clinics involved Bikram. Someone would demonstrate the posture while Bikram would say the words. The trainees would take notes. Over time, those notes were typed up and distributed to classmates.

As Diane gave us a little history, I could tell she was anything but timid. I could also tell she was going to teach a fierce class and, frankly, the nipple pain was wearing me out. I tried to grab a place in the back row, but, good Ganesh, those spots get grabbed first. Diane's class seemed to fly by. And the best part—she pretty much said the Dialogue verbatim. Yay! It was great to hear it done, and yet done in her own style. I realized librarian was all wrong for her—she'd be a great auctioneer. She's got an entrenched New England accent and she rat-a-tats the words, it almost sounds like she says, "Balancing Stick, do I hear $500? I've got $500, do I hear $600, $600, $600, $600, going, going, going, gone!"

After Diane's romping class, time for our final posture clinic. Spine Twist. Posture #26. This is it, we are here at the end of the yellow brick road.

I had made up my mind that I was not going to end with a whimper. I started this process with Bikram offering his microphone to me and, be damned, I was not about to fizzle at the end and crawl out with my tail between my legs.

Plus which, Spine Twist is a little stink bomb at the end of the road. The floor series postures are, by nature, a bit shorter than the standing series and they seemed to have rolled a bit more easily. Spine Twist involves a lot of lefts and rights and so I studied my little heart out this past weekend.

There's a new gal behind the clipboard, Lynn. She reminds me of Minnie Driver – the one with the curly hair who was in Good Will Hunting. Her face is rounder and her hair is super short. Nonetheless, she looks friendly.

I got up there, and I must admit, I rocked the house. I'm doing great and the Dialogue instructs us to spell the word heel, actually spell it out, haitch ee ee ell. I'm pleased with my verbatim-ness, I spell the word heel and I hear some titters and I figure Mili is snickering at me struggling to bang out every word and then, I'm not sure why, but I spell the word knee and then the crowd is cackling, people are holding their sides, honestly, I feel a bit rattled, I'm not sure what is so damn funny.

I lose my train of thought for, I don't know, 7 or 10 seconds but then, no, I remind myself that I'm Scottish and American Indian, a Taurus born in the year of the Dragon, they don't make 'em any more stubborn than me.

I realign the word train and I get to the last line, the very last line about the spine being stacked up like a pearl necklace and, kerplooey!, the words vanish. I know I need to bring it on home, but I also know I should not improvise at all, so I "borrow" the words from the other side Dialogue. And I'm so pleased, so very pleased.

I turn to face Lynn behind the clipboard. I do expect her comments to be about 30 percent rating the final posture and then the remaining 70 percent wrapping up where I've been and where I'll go and final wise-older-teacher kind of pat on the head.

She shakes her head side to side, as if she's saying "no, no, no" over and over again. Her head re-centers and her steely gray eyes bore into my eyes.

In a flinty voice, she says, "Drop the comedy act. With that funny business, I can guarantee, you will not last at any studio for more than three or four weeks."

The room collectively takes a stiff inhale on this news. We all didn't see it coming. Lynn senses this and I sense she'll clarify, or, better yet, retract.

"Well, maybe you could last up to six weeks if there were a teacher shortage and the studio was desperate."

She continued, saying that I'm not to improvise at all and so I try to defend my honor as best I can, saying that I had borrowed from the Dialogue for the other side. She snarks that that isn't my job; besides which, what will I do when I get to the other side and I've already used up those words?

She hits me with I think is quite a rabbit punch: "Strong teachers will always go to the Dialogue; weak ones will stray."

And to always remember: there is zero room in the yoga studio for any kind of humor.

(Really? See, now, I couldn't disagree more. Bikram is funny. Rajashree tells funny stories. Craig barked like a dog once in class. Emmy—okay, Emmy is pretty serious.)

I suppose it is my fault, I did have fairly specific expectations about my final posture clinic, that it would be fun and we'd be dancing silly dances and high-fiving each other. At no point in my scenario did I expect to hear that I wouldn't last a month.

I sat down next to Mili. She and I have had this running joke that every time I add a word, I owe her five dollars. I sit down, and I feel like I'm about to cry. Mili leans over and whispers, "Naughty naughty, you added like mad. I think you owe me at least 20 dollars."

I went into the bathroom and cried and could not stop the weeping. I was sad that it was coming to an end and sad that Mili lives so far away, morose that I'll probably never see her again.

Mili finds me hunched over a sink, sobbing, and explains the raucous laughter.

Turns out that when I spelled the word heel, I spelled it: haitch ee ell ell—hell. So the snickering started. But when I spelled the word knee, I went phonetic: en ee ee ee.

I'll just ask Lynn tomorrow what her intent was with her notes to me. Perhaps she didn't intend to shred my tired little ego. It is possible she thought she was oozing kindness. Doubtful, but possible.

Yok scolds me on the way home. Haven't I heard? This Lynn woman is a very high-ranking Bikram teacher. Rumor has it Bikram calls Lynn for advice on who to graduate. I tell Yok I cannot fathom that Bikram would allow people to be mean to each other. Yok teased me about that Cobra situation yesterday—wasn't he being mean? No, no, he exudes kindness.

Yok says that maybe Lynn just doesn't like me.

I admit I am a love/hate kind of person—but who could decide in less than two minutes to hate me so very much?

Cannot believe it is time to pack up already. The exciting bit is that we finished the Dialogue a week early. Some prior teacher trainings have gone so pokey, they've had to stay up and do posture clinic until the wee hours, just to get done in time for graduation. Craig said tonight we'd most likely have time next week to actually teach mock classes, more than one posture at a time. That would be great experience.

We have a lecture tomorrow night that starts at eleven at night! Some biochemist dude who has proven somethingorother about biochemistry and yoga postures. Sounds interesting; just wish it were a tad earlier. We actually lobbied heavily for a midnight class in lieu of the Saturday morning fun. Craig vetoed that idea.

SATURDAY 4 JUNE

# of days in yoga boot camp: 55
# of days until graduation: 7

The stiffness has gone to a point of absurdity. I now need to wait for the handicapped bathroom. I can sit down okay by myself in under a minute. But getting back up off the toilette—no can do. Those handicapped railings are my saving grace.

My head is cooling, a little, about that "you won't last a month" Lynn woman. Not cool yet, but maybe Yok is right, maybe smiling and saying nothing is the way to go here. Maybe after I graduate, I'll drop her a note. I'm not quite sure what I'll say, but I do think she shouldn't be mean. Not with a week to go.

The guest biochemist guy started late, but was finally finished around one in the morning. Snuck in about four hours of sleep, then up again for our final Craig class.

I do know I felt quite morally vindicated this morning. Our last Craig class, and he spelled heel and knee. I swear I heard him spelling knee the way I did en ee ee eee. Hoorah! Great minds think (and spell) alike.

Had just enough time for a smoothie from across the street.

Then—CPR certification from 10:00 A.M. until 5:00 P.M. Awfully gamey and tired, don't really know how I did it.

TUESDAY 7 JUNE

# of days in yoga boot camp: 58
# of days until graduation: 4

Top-o-the-news: CBS 60 Minutes will air a segment on Bikram tomorrow night, June 8. The air feels electrified, the way it does backstage, right before the curtain goes up and a prop goes missing and a fuse blows and the audience claps.

I'm utterly lousy with a cold/bronchitis thing. Almost stayed in the back row this morning; I simply couldn't fathom making it all the way through class. Actually, when I woke up with a fever this morning, I did seriously consider calling the mothership and asking if I could please have a sick day. Then I remember: I will leave only by stretcher.

Mili convinced me to come with her to the third row. And there were her other Aussie friends—Michael the chiropractor and his precious wife Susan. Mili said it would feel like home, to be surrounded by friends and yet there wouldn't be any of the first row pressure. Plus which, they'd all send me healing powers.

Had an awful teacher. Can't remember his name, but he held us in Pada Hastasana for about 17 minutes and the class ran well over 2 hours and me and my cold and my slime-filled lungs did not need someone on some kind of podium power trip. The shivering thing was only enhanced by the fever.

I sleep after the morning class and, for the first time, I curl up and sleep during the afternoon mock class. Lynn was again behind the clipboard. I figured if she caught me napping and yelled at me then I'd remind her I'm just here for show. If I won't last three weeks, in her mind, no sense in my wasting her precious resources on people that can be saved.

I feel a little guilty about the mid-class nap. Then I remind myself what Prince always says: the body wouldn't ask for the sleep if it didn't need it. Gosh I miss Prince.

(Note to self: you have 70 hours 'til Prince. Shave legs. Condition. Pluck.)

For the evening class, I decide to return to the front row. Mili cautions against it. I tell her I feel at home up there with my neighborhood. Plus which, it is a great spot to rest because you are snugged up against the podium and very few people can see if you've gone down. And I do have every intention of resting a lot. I do believe my fever is higher and everything seems to be worsening.

Faroh, a guy from India, is teaching. Bikram decides he will take the class as a student. He puts his mat behind my mat. I think about moving, but then, man, would that be an insult. Maybe, like last week, he'll sense my weakness and leave me alone.

I start class feeling like a rock star. I had all my mat toys lined up and ready to go: lip balm, Cold-eze, Zicam, throat lozenges, Advil. My neighbors promise to send lots of energy and despite the reduced lung capacity and the fever, I was feeling the healing love of yoga.

Bikram left me alone at the beginning. Phew! So relieved; maybe he'll just focus on his postures and I'll focus on mine.

False confidence.

(Put another way: what the hell was I thinking? My only defense is that the fever must have produced delusions.)

Right after our water break, which we fondly call party time, in Standing Head to Knee, Bikram whispers, "Lock your damn knee. Miss Pink, how many times I have to tell you?"

I decided to ignore him entirely. Quite naughty behavior, talking in class. And clearly he was in some kind of bad mood that had nothing to do with my wobbly knee.

Maybe that was my lesson to be learned with the crazy Calcutta contortionist. I had let him steal my peace. No more.

I did pretty well.

Standing Bow: "Psst. What da hell is that Miss Pink? You aren't even kicking."

Balancing Stick: "Psst. You hear me, I know you do. Terrible Balancing Stick. Fix your arms. Raise your foot. You are lazy Miss Pink."

We get to Triangle and I'm quite mad.

"Psst. Miss Pink, that Triangle is a piece of shit bullshit posture."

So I turned around and asked him, what do I need to do? Step wider? Lunge more? And I cannot believe what comes sliding out of my mouth, skittering out of control, like a car sliding down an icy hill in the dark of December.

"I'm sorry Boss, I just don't think 'piece of shit' is very instructional for me."

TRIKANASANA
TRIANGLE

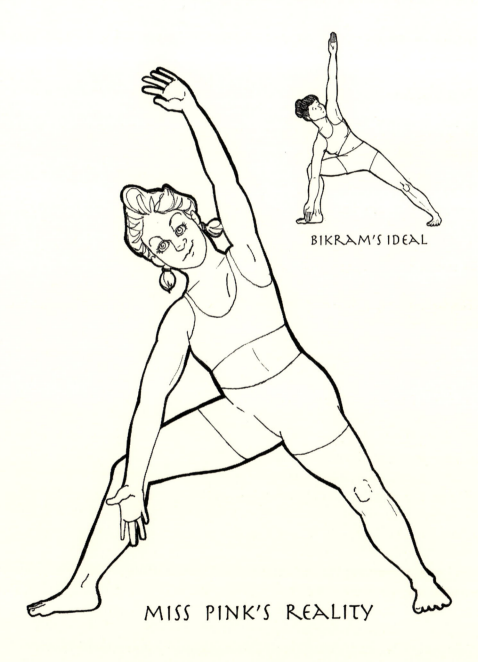

BIKRAM'S IDEAL

MISS PINK'S REALITY

Oh my god, help me, I will be carried out on a stretcher. I haven't meant to sass my new false idol, but, honestly, he's been saying the same thing over and over again and clearly someone needs to change tactics. I won't name names, but the one who needs to change has a topknot on the top of his head.

He nods, he doesn't look angry.

He stands directly behind me, and puts one foot in between my two legs, like he is preparing to perform a Heimlich. His right foot slides out and steps on my right thigh biceps. He's saying "seeet down alllll the way." His angry little heel starts banging on my right thigh bicep like a ball peen hammer.

"No, no, Miss Pink, your hip came up. Hip goes down. Look in the mirror."

I look to the mirror to see what he's talking about because I feel as though my crotch is about to plunk flat on the floor, that's how far down I feel. And I'm glad he told me to look, I feel as though the mirror will defend me and my posture.

He grabs my chin and flips it back around.

"No, no, look with your eyessssssss Miss Pink. Not your head, your eyes."

His right heel has slithered around to my left hip and is banging insistently on my left hipbone, trying to push it back, I think. His left hand is stretching my left hand up and his right hand is attempting, without any success, to convince my right thigh to go lower.

He concludes our semiprivate lesson with, "You remember this, yes, do perfect second set?"

And I don't know what I replied. I was thinking to myself, well, now, this is quite odd and intimate and everything really hurts and if we were in a grocery store, him pulling off his shenanigans, wrapping a foot around my waist, we'd be arrested for indecency. What would my nice Lutheran cake-baking (deceased) grandmother say if she saw this?

By Standing Separate Leg Head to Knee, I thought I was out of the danger zone.

"You do not need to bend your knee, Miss Pink. Just tuck your chin in more, and roll, like rabbit, tuck your damn chin."

I cannot tuck. When I tuck, I get winking fireflies dancing in front of me and then some phlegm comes rolling up and I cannot breathe through my nose because it no longer is functioning as an oxygen distribution system, it is too clogged, it is really there, the nose, to be about symmetry and decoration.

He throws some pebbles from the floor at me. Then stands up and I think, ruh-roh, the crazy Calcutta contortionist is going to start humping my leg and he says "Oooo, you make me so mad." He stomps away, feet pounding into the floor, and I do imagine that steam is blowing out of his ears, like Yosemite Sam, only with less clothing.

Well, I think, at least he's gone and I can rest now, lay out a few postures.

Bikram returns after Wind Removing Pose. He doesn't say anything to me, he just gets on his mat and does his posture and I do my posture and I'm glad we have come to an understanding.

I do a fairly decent Cobra and he starts in again with it being awful.

He's on a warpath now, this is no longer our private little battle. He tells everyone that can hear him to stop class so that they can see Miss Pink's "piece of shit Cobra."

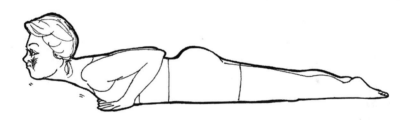

So I go up, admittedly more garden snake than Cobra—but the Dialogue is very clear on this point: use 100 percent spine strength, no help from the arms. So I use my arms a wee bit and he's yelling at me and he demands to know what I'm thinking and I say that I can't come up with my hands and he gets all Yosemite Sam on me and says use your damn hands, use your damn hands.

I say, "The Dialogue says no hands and I will not cheat."

He looks murderous.

"Miss Pink, you not using your body at all. You are the only person in this room that gets fatter and fatter every day; every day I come in to teach you and your body is bigger. Why? Because you are not working at all, you are lying on the floor, your mind is on vacation."

I wonder if he's referencing my humming of the burger song. Because, oh yeah, that was a little break for the mind. More of like a long lunch break, though, than out-and-out holiday.

Bikram grabs the microphone from Faroh, the teacher.

Faroh chuckles and looks down at me with compassion in his eyes and says, "You are in the wrong place today."

Bikram is fueled by frustration, he can barely contain himself.

"Look at her. Miss Pink, she's not doing anything. Absolutely nothing. Wasting her time. You should see her every posture, she's minus 10,000 percent. She's not using her body. So her body is not getting anything. That is why she has the same body, a big fat junk body.

She is not going inside, bones to skin, hair to toes. She's only doing what she can do very comfortably, easy way, like a feather touching the body. She's not using the body even one percent. I know, all the postures, I watch her.

If you have a student like that, you have to kill them. And if they don't listen, throw them out of your class. You do not want to have a reputation of having bad students.

I have to tell the truth, she's just floating on the top of the water with floaters."

Floaters seems like a very American word for Bikram. Strikes me as an odd word choice. Then again, I remember that he always says he has never learned to swim, so perhaps he is well acquainted with inflatable armbands. That's a very funny mental picture, actually, watermelon-colored floaters on the King of Yogis.

"Go ahead, do the posture, do Cobra."

Crap. He's still talking to me. Right? I mean he's still there and I'm still here and I do resent the thing about getting fat every day. Because, honestly, that is an electrolyte issue.

"She has an ugly Cobra but I know she can do much better."

No, see, that's nice. He can be compassionate.

"I have never met anybody so lazy mentally. Go ahead. Go. Use the Dialogue. It says to use your hands. Elbows at a 90-degree angle. So go up. Come up. More up. Keep going. How do you feel now?"

I mutter something about, oh, yeah, I'm feeling groovy.

"How many billion times you heard if you cannot go up, use your hand strength, go up until your bellybutton is pressing into the floor."

Honestly—the man is quite stubborn. I mention, again, that there is honestly zero Dialogue pertaining to use of hands in Cobra. I'm only doing as his Dialogue says.

His eyes squint into little diamond slits.

"Okay, how about Triangle? How about Awkward? Every single posture are you going to explain to me why you are not doing it?"

I don't have an answer for that. Well, I do, actually. I have lots of questions. Like in Triangle, he always says to keep my elbow at my knee but then he tells me to put my fingers in between my toes and if I do that, then my elbow is below my knee. So what's up with that? And Awkward, well, I've made great strides with that posture.

"You know what? Your brain is somewhere in Mexico. Or Timbuktu, wherever that is."

He hands the microphone back to Faroh, who mightily regains control of the class and we do Locust pose. I will admit, I have felt really stymied by this one. Everyone but me has legs that fly through the air with the greatest of ease.

SALABHASANA
LOCUST

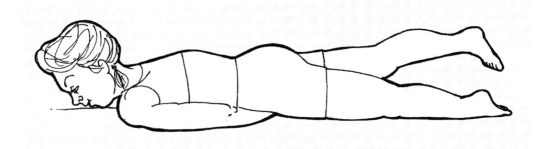

MISS PINK'S REALITY
BIKRAM'S IDEAL

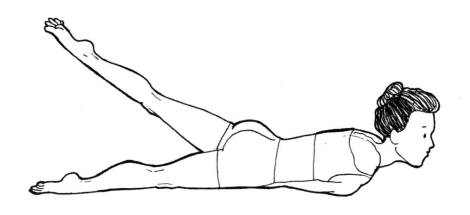

He comes up beside me and starts again.

"Your foot only comes up off the floor one inch or two inches, what is wrong with you? Use your hands, use the other leg, use your shoulders, get everything up off the floor."

I hate to bring up the deficiencies of his precious Dialogue, but there is zero instruction about using my other leg. So I say this, I try to be meek, I say, listen, when my right leg is in the air, then the left leg is relaxed and easy, on vacation.

"Who tell you that? I never say that. Use your damn leg."

Really? The floor leg?

"Are you an idiot? Yes, yes, use the other leg, you'll see big difference."

And, oh my gosh, my leg flew through the air. Wow. That was pretty inspiring.

"Better Miss Pink. Now, for both legs, use your goddamn hands."

And I did. And then Faroh said he'd help and everyone started cheering and, wow, it felt totally different to me and I could just tell my legs were up off the floor.

I put my right ear on the towel, proper Savasana. I want so much to cry. I can see all sorts of heads popping up, like whack-a-mole, little heads rising everywhere and lots of people are winking and smiling at me and giving me thumbs-up. Even Jaunty Hat Jamie props herself up on her elbows, givbes me a thumbs-up and whispers "doing great!" I want so much for a phlegmy boohoo, the kind that makes you feel sick in the middle but better in the end.

But, oh no, I will not cry in front of this man.

I haven't left the room and he is still there, though he has sat back down on his mat. I think of all the postures, I am most sloppy and most uninspired in Full Locust.

POORNA SALABHASANA
FULL LOCUST

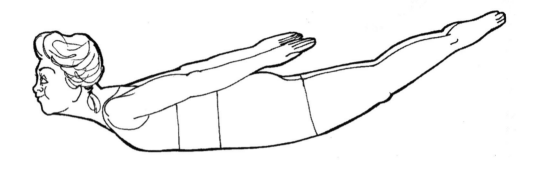

MISS PINK'S REALITY
BIKRAM'S IDEAL

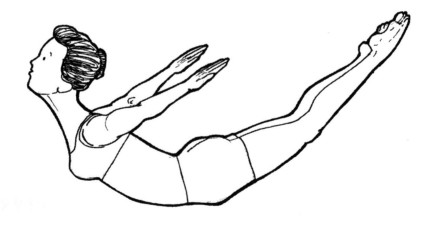

I don't know why, but I did feel that I had to exercise some kind of stiff upper lipness. I turn around and find a splinter-sized bit of dignity and I say to Bikram, "Listen, boss, just so there'll be no surprises, I hate this posture, this my worst one, worse than all of the others. And I'm tired and I am not going to even give it 85 percent energy—just so you know."

He smiled a sweet little smile and suddenly I notice a winking glimmer in his beady eyes and he pats me on my leg and says, "You are good, Miss Pink. I know you can do good."

Things seem clearer now. Is he actually trying to tell me that he knows more about me than I do? I suppose after four decades of teaching yoga, he's got a few extra tricks up his sleeve. I scanned his eyes one more time for venom or disgust and all I was saw was love. Love in a breathtaking raw pure form.

As I gather up whatever strength I have, he's smiling. And as I plunge headlong into my most-hated posture, he's leaning forward and cheering for me and giving small pointers, whispering "chin up more, one inch more" and "kick a little harder" and I'm half-expecting Jekyl/Hyde to grab the microphone again and find new ways to add to my shame. He leans forward, and says again, more softly, "You did good Miss Pink. Very good." And he gives my calf muscle a squeeze and I feel stronger and I feel loved and I feel like everything will be okay.

I manage to stay in the room the rest of the class and I do manage to not cry in front of him.

When I entered the locker room, I realized that my Miss Pink identity was no longer a secret. All kinds of hugs and all kinds of comments, ranging from "I'm so glad us fat girls have a role model" to "don't worry, the weight will come off" to "hang in there."

Adi motioned for me to come to her and she starts telling me about her Bikram mentor, the teacher that inspired her and that her teacher was overweight like me and that her teacher had just died. Today. Yesterday alive. Today dead. And then she just sort of looked at me like—the moral of this story is? And I don't know, I felt awful for her loss but I didn't need another reason to cry and I'm not fat. It is electrolyte imbalances!

I finally escape the hugging gauntlet and, borrowing a trick from Shannon, grab a stack of towels and go into the furthest stall and shriek and cry and scream, towels muting my anguished, pitiful little sounds. I want to go home. I want (weirdly) Jell-O with whipped cream and my sheep jammies and soft 600-count sheets and Prince and my kitten purring on the small of my back.

But there is no escaping, not tonight.

Tonight is the talent show.

Which, ironically, involves me reading a section from my book about how all the TV people told me I was too fat.

I was actually nervous. This is the first time reading my book out loud to nonfamily people. Well, okay, they are my family now. But it is a big and diverse crowd. I think my divorce travails are slightly funny, but you never know. Plus which, Bikram and Rajashree are to be seated in the front row. And, I'm having doubts. Amy and Mili and Yok all convinced me this would be great—writing is my talent. It is my favorite thing to do, for sure. But still, maybe this is not the right venue.

Bikram and Rajashree were there in the front row. They looked like your average married couple who had just had a giant fight and still had to come to some dumb social engagement. I looked at them once; Bikram looked madder than I'd ever seen and Rajashree looked like she had won the argument and yet was still mad as she couldn't believe he would have the audacity to say that idiotic thing he said.

Here's the section I read, from Leaving the Land of Should:

22 June 2001

Just got off the phone. E*Trade insists they'll hire me by Labor Day. Which would be wonderful comeuppance. Crazy Bloomberg bastard. Snotty CNN cretins. I suppose I should be flattered that CNN thought I was evening anchor material. Slightly insane that they think I can lose 40 pounds in 6 weeks. Well, I mean, I could pull that off, I suppose. But they also want breast implants and facial liposuction—I called around, I can't even get an appointment in the next six months. Plus which, even if I had my fat little face vacuumed tomorrow, isn't six weeks a short recovery time?

I'm doing my meditation stuff but it still seems like the universe is making sure my ego keeps getting little rabbit punches along the way.

Like today. It started off like any normal kind of day. Get up, mop up greyhound urine off the kitchen floor, shower, get ready for the big Bloomberg interview.

It is with Bloomberg Radio, which is a step down from television. But if I can nail the job, then I can leave my annoying, overweight, flatulent, impotent husband.

I was told the interview was merely a formality—the current morning host specifically requested they hire me.

We do the formalities and then Ivan the Interviewer asks me, "Which is stronger, the dollar or the yen?"

What a silly question. Jeesh. I hide my annoyance and ask Ivan to clarify—stronger how—relative to each other or relative to the euro? Stronger over what time frame?

Ivan says he didn't expect me to be one of those detail-oriented journalists. He puts finger quotes around the word journalist. I do not like finger quoters, they are passive-aggressive. Besides, this is financial news, not Entertainment Tonight.

He then says that he's sorry, but my weight is an issue. I'm confused—I'm too fat for radio? Ivan says they will film the radio show—sort of the way Howard Stern films his show—and so, sorry, but the new trend in television is the heroin-chic look and I simply won't do.

I am loathe to mix personal with business ... but I tell a small, teensy lie and say that my husband has been laid off and I need the job.

Ivan claims he sympathizes and offers me a position in the mailroom as a file clerk that pays 28,000 a year. Quite a far cry from my prior six-figure salary.

I'm dazed. I'm thinking "poor file clerk" "rich wife" "poor file clerk" "rich wife" and I really wish that there was a third choice and I sniff and say that I'm awful at filing and I appreciate the opportunity and there you go.

Thinking it isn't possible for my day to get worse—in fact, walking down Park Avenue, tulips a-bloom, sun shining, I say to myself, "Could this day get any worse?" It does.

I have dinner with husband Ken and his new boss Hans. Ken introduces me and Hans asks, "What do you do?" and before I could say "I'm in television" or "I'm the NASDAQ girl", ohgodhelpme, Ken said "My wife? Why, she's a great little decorator." I look alarmed and Ken clarifies. "Well, to be fair—she's a great decorator and an all-around fabulous homemaker."

After a tortuously long dinner, I tear into Ken.

Decorator?! Homemaker?

Ken actually cries and admits that he has "wife envy"—that Hans's wife is an uber wife. She is an economist and a bond trader. She sleeps a mere three hours a night and has thrown herself into renovating their 150-year-old country cottage. She's such an astonishing specimen of a wife that when the cottage fireplace had smoke damage, uber-wife took a yearlong architectural history class to learn about mantles of the cottage's era and then went to masonry school and learned how to carve marble so she could then make a mantle from scratch.

Ken says when we married, he just assumed I should become that kind of uber-wife.

I get pissy, I don't care that he's crying, these are the first tears I've seen him shed in over a decade—but, honestly, for 15 years he has watched me struggle with microwaving frozen dinners but he has the gall to introduce me as a homemaker?

I'm on this tirade, this brilliant monologue and it just tumbles out. "I will not stay married to you. I will not stay married to you. I've put up with your gassy colon and your aversion to deodorant and your mother and your toenail fungus. You are a diary snooper and I will not be the wife of a smelly snooper. No. Not for eight more times I won't."

I felt bitchy adding in that last bit, the eight more times thing, but he knew. Oh, he knew!

Two months ago, he had read my diary when I was visiting my mum. The entry he read—and then ripped out—was the part where I was trying to quantify our sex life.

We had made love twice in seven years. Our marital relations average, therefore, was once every one thousand two hundred and seventy-seven days.

We should stay married thirty more years. That would imply we would make love eight point six more times by my seventieth birthday.

Perhaps sexual deprivation leads to insanity. Feels like it. On the very day that Bloomberg doesn't work out, on the very day that I reject a job offer—a subpar one, no doubt—I shout to the man that pays the bills that I no longer want to be married.

Ken looks pale, his freckles fade, he's shocked. (Of course he's surprised, because uber-wives don't leave marriages. Though if I were truly an uber-wife, I would go to paper-making school to make my own divorce decree paper and then go to law school to file my own papers on the paper I milled by hand.)

He then weeps like a hungry child who lost his mommy at the mall food court. He's genuinely surprised. He finally pulls himself together and says he'll set me free while I still have a few good years left.

I ask what that means, the few good years left thing.

He goes right to how hard it is being married to a writer who always harps on word choice. It didn't come out right—what he meant to say was that at age thirty-seven, I'm not exactly a looker.

I ask what the hell that means, the looker thing.

He says I'm doing the word thing again, and that all he did mean was that he wouldn't oppose the divorce. As a quick added potshot, he quips that writers should be able to use more words than the "thing" thing that I use.

I am relieved and then he keeps talking, he says he's sorry we didn't have the sex life I wanted, he just wished I had told him, he had no crystal ball, he had no way of knowing that sex was that important to go at it more than once a year.

I get angrier, he's so clever to make it my fault, see how easily he did that?

He says I haven't exactly improved with age, the trend isn't good, so let's do a quick divorce so I stand a chance of nabbing someone before I fully morph into a hairy crone.

I tell him that men are drawn to me the same way he's drawn to a Philadelphia cheese steak, moth to flame, that when I'm eighty, my college-age pool boy will be desperate to get his mitts on me.

That all I've ever wanted was to be happy and I will be happy if it kills me.

And then he says he had no idea I was so full of myself, so vain, so conceited. And he also says he had no idea I was so obsessed with this being happy thing.

He put finger quotes around the word happy. I cannot stay married to someone who puts finger quotes around happy, like it is an abstract concept, a figment solely of my imagination.

I close my eyes and I envision my divorce court. It will look like it does on Ally McBeal, dark mahogany paneling, tall bench for the judge, green leather swively chairs. And the judge will be nice and jolly and kind, like John Lithgow.

And when Judge Lithgow asks me for the reason for the divorce, I'm going with that. I'm not going to be dull and say, "the marriage is irretrievably broken."

Oh no, I'm going to look the judge in the eye and I will say, "Your honor, the reason for this divorce is finger quotes around the word happy."

23 June 2001

By morning, we were too tired to be mad.

We mapped out a plan. There are some things I cannot fix. I told Ken that I'd work on my own self-esteem situation and he should pick on one of his issues to work on. Between the anger at his mother, the fact that his family hates me, the fact that he's adopted, or the fact that he's sad about being diabetic—just pick one and stare at it and try to find a way to work on it. He wants me to "assign" him a topic. No thanks, I'm not a marble-carver nor am I a topic-picker. I tell him to select one issue and just go nutso on it. Not fix it, but stare into the belly of the beast.

Join an adoption support group, find a nutritionist, read a book on diabetes, journal about his childhood—anything that will make him feel better. He says he'll pick his own topic and it'll be a surprise.

I'm not sure he'll really do anything. Actually, I am secretly hoping he'll do nothing. I feel so good announcing that I want o-u-t. I don't want to take it back. I feel like I can breathe again.

I could not have survived this without wise-yoda-counselor friend Tom. Tom rallied Dennis (husband of Barbara) and the two of them took me out drinking—naturally, Ken had to work. Saturday night, and he has to work. Tom and Dennis and I throw darts and drink cider and I can't remember where the really good dart bar is located and we are driving in circles and I get out my cell phone to call Ken and Dennis snatches it from me and says "You need to cut the ties. Don't let him know you need him." And I felt like I was me again, Tom and Dennis made me remember who I used to be, I felt like I had awakened from the GoodWifeComa.

Forty-eight hours after the Great I Want Out Proclamation, I got stung badly by a giant thumb-sized bumblebee. I got swollen and weird feeling and Ken came to the rescue and I thought, as he applied paste to the sting area, I can't leave this. (Though he kept rubbing the paste in a circle around the sting—not straight on top of the sting—and we had an odd did-not/did-too argument about paste application. Swear to god, one day, I'll drag that man to an eye doctor. He's never been. Says it is all a sham, everyone that ever goes comes home with glasses, so if you don't need glasses, then don't go to an eye doctor.)

So we are semi-arguing about bee paste application and I feel dizzy and I'm glad he's there. Maybe my mum is right, this is a rough patch, we'll find our way back to each other.

Everyone really liked it! I got laughter in weird places. Like, the part about the uber wife who carved her own mantle—entirely true!—and I had to stop for a few seconds to let the laughter die down. Go figure.

I was swarmed in the hallway and in the bathroom, people wanting to know when it would be published.

Called Prince when I got home. I told him every detail of today's public drubbing. So often, people assume that just because I'm sort of sassy and brazen, that I can brook anything from anyone. Not true. Not true at all!

Then the tear spigot blew its top and I cried and mewled into the phone until three in the morning. I want so very much to be at home. I really really really don't want to be here any more.

WEDNESDAY 8 JUNE

# of days in yoga boot camp: 59
# of days until graduation: 3
# of hours til Prince arrives: 46

Couldn't have asked for a more perfect day. I mean, if I were a scriptwriter and the director gave me carte blanche, I would have never dreamed up this scenario.

Good morning class. Two hours long—and breathing was hard—but I could feel a lot of the postures working better after last night's, ahem, private class with Bikram. The cold had worsened, which seemed unfathomable to me, that it could get worse. But it did.

By afternoon I'm so very bone-weary. I didn't get a chance for my afternoon nap. And the only food that even sounds remotely palatable is (bizarrely) Diet Coke and pickles and watermelon.

I need to talk to Craig. I had an absurd question about Dialogue, but I want something from him. I think I want a day off. A less-hot class. Tea and sympathy. Jell-O and canned pears. Honestly, I wanted some good old-fashioned there-there pity. And sleep. But definitely a get-out-of-jail-for-free card.

I'm waiting and I'm waiting and someone in front of me has usurped every molecule from Craig. A very nice staffer from the front desk floats up and says that it appears Craig is a bit tied up—is there anything she can help me with?

I start crying, giant tears bursting out sideways and I murble through my phlegmy chest and on-fire throat that if Bikram is going to withhold my teaching certificate due to my allegedly bad Triangle posture, that I'd like to know it now so I can go home and nap and eat Cool Whip.

She squeezes my hand and looks deeply into my eyes and asks, "Can you hang in there for just two more days?"

And I say no. It is my first defeat in ages. No. I know there's no stretcher involved (though my ego would beg to differ; the ego remains in intensive care) but I honestly cannot stay. She squeezes my hand and assures me that I'll be fine.

The good news is, Bikram is not teaching tonight. Rumor has it he has gone out of town.

Fine. I proudly plunk my mat down front and center—directly in front of the podium. It is a favorite spot of mine. There's no mirror to look at, so it is a refreshing way to focus on the feeling of each posture, instead of relying on visual cues. And I'm right next to Emily, so if the going gets tough, I can replay my Swan Lake ballerina fantasy.

Damn. The best laid plans of mats and men...

Right as I'm feeling cozy in my mat placement, the King of Yogi's staff arrives and prepares his throne. First, his favorite orange and pink towel that says "Hot Stuff" is stretched across the white podium chair. Wrinkles are smoothed. Next, someone comes in with a blue Seattle Space Needle mug with hot chai tea. Often a third person comes in and readjusts the placement of the chai and places a black headband next to the chai and re-smooths the Hot Stuff towel, to be certain there are no wrinkles.

Adi and Shannon and Mili and Dallas Julie all come over to express concern that I should maybe move my mat and avoid Bikram. Mili offers up space in her third row neighborhood. Firefighter Charlie and Strawberry Julie give me a pat and a thumbs-up.

You know what? Maybe I've overdosed on ZiCam and Zinc, but I'm thinking, bring it on Bendyboy. First off, I don't think that telling me my posture is "bullshit" is the way to teach properly. And secondly, if he is some giant yogi teacher maestro, then clearly he has failed me. Thirdly, I paid my money to come here and I have no intention of hiding.

I'm shocked. Right at the beginning, he sets the tone.

Right there, first set of Pranayama Breathing, "Good, now, elbows up more Miss Pink." He sounds nice and warm.

At Half Moon, he points to Pigtail Sarah and says "Come down just like her. Miss Pink, you are as good as her. I know this."

We get to Triangle, we gaze at each other like cowboys preparing for a sunset showdown.

He starts the conversation.

"Now. Miss Pink, your Triangle is all wrong. It is worse than last night I think!"

He laughs and I think he winks. I feel it is his olive branch, our own little mea culpa.

I reply "You have to tell me how to do it right, word by word."

He takes me through every step. For starters, my stance was too wide and sometimes, with shorter people, narrower feet can be a big help.

I attempt the sitting all the way down thing, but both hips have giant cramps in them, like toe cramps only 17 times more vicious.

He remains displeased, frowning, shaking his head. I remain insistent, I'm staring right at him, I do mean business, I will not leave this smelly inferno until we do it right.

He announces to the class to take a break, as Miss Pink will do her own personal third set of Triangle.

The whole class starts to cheer for me, which revives my just-back-from-the-ICU ego. I sit all the way down and I have tears running down my face, it hurts so bad, I do honestly think it hurts worse than cracked kneecaps.

I say, quietly, "It really hurts Boss" and he nods compassionately and says, "I know, Miss Pink, I know. Yoga is supposed to hurt!"

On his instruction, one class mate grabs ahold of my left hand and keeps pulling it up towards the ceiling and then another classmate pulls my right hand all the way down to the floor and then, wow, my shoulders are opening and I don't think I'm imagining it, but my phlegmy lungs feel quite clear all of the sudden.

I start to slide a bit, Bikram instructs another student to get their foot up there to stop mine from slipping. Then the guy pulling the right hand down gently nudges my right knee back with his spare hand.

In a flash, I understand that I've gotten the Friends for Life thing all wrong. It isn't that one person needs to be appointed to be my friend. It is that this entire group, they are all friends and they will all stay with me through the dawn of time and, again, I want to weep plishy happy tears.

Bikram looks quite pleased.

"Now that, Miss Pink, is perfect. You now have the best Triangle in the whole class, probably even whole world. Now then, do your own Triangle, other side."

He's grinning like a proud poppa and between my wincing, I'm trying hard to smile up at him to show him that I am grateful that we are coming to an end with this battle.

TRIKANASANA
TRIANGLE

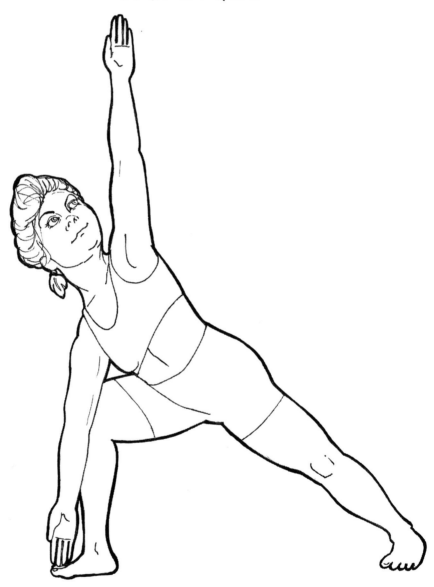

MISS PINK'S (NEW & IMPROVED) REALITY

Next posture, Standing Separate Leg Head to Knee he says, "Miss Pink, you have a very perfectly well-proportioned body. Use your proportions to your advantage and put your weight fooooorrrward." Oh, yeah! Now that felt quite different.

Now this feels fun. Painful, yes, but somehow a good kind of pain and my nose is actually clearing. Yoga curing the common cold? Perhaps. Each posture we take time and I ask questions and I realized that so many of my issues were misinterpretations of the Dialogue and I do vow, on that sweat-soaked sisal, that I will never, ever, ever change the Dialogue.

At the end of class, as he is breezing out of the room, I tap his ankle. He stops and looks at me, almost harshly.

I do a quick bow to him with my hands in prayer, he has so wowed me, I did not know it was possible to respect and admire someone so much. I say quickly "Thank you very much."

He shakes his chin a couple of times quickly, as though he's got water in his ears. And then he leaves and I feel like a fool, there's probably some guru etiquette thing. Wait—there's that thing about not touching the guru, right? Damn.

***

We get our dinner break—followed by a nice cherry on top. Bikram has arranged for giant televisions in the yoga studio room and we are all to watch the 60 Minutes segment. I'll admit I was worried. Sometimes Bikram goes off on these odd halfcocked sentiments that, if taken out of context, could make him sound—well—a bit zany.

It was perfect. He looked great and the piece ran about 20 minutes. They traveled back to Calcutta and there were people lining the streets to wave to him. He had great answers for everything.

"You have a lot of money."

"Yes. I do like money. Yogis don't have to be poor."

"This is almost like McYoga—you know, like McDonald's."

"Good. I like McDonald's. Good fries."

His evening lecture meandered for a bit, it didn't seem to have the same storytelling sway to it as other lectures. I was just about to get up to slip out to the bathroom when he asked, "Where is Miss Pink?"

So I waved and regretted not having left five minutes earlier.

He started out by saying, "Miss Pink, she does not cry. I beat the crap out of her yesterday, you all remember? I tell her bullshit things, I say she's ugly, she's fat, she's old, nothing, she will not cry. Your eyes were red, right Miss Pink? But did you cry?"

No boss, not during class.

"Miss Pink rock solid. Now, most people be mad and pissed off and say fuck you Bikram. But what does she say? She say thank you Bikram. She thanked me. Miss Pink win, I lose." And then he bowed to me.

For nearly two hours, he talked at length about our battles. His frustration with me. How awfully hard it was to convey to me, an allegedly intelligent woman, how much the postures needed to be fixed. We must, as yoga teachers, learn to be good and patient teachers to all students, "even if their postures look as bad as Miss Pink's."

Oddly, in the middle of the nice-fest, he caught David the Lamppost nodding off in a corner. (It was hot and muggy and, quite frankly, if he hadn't been talking about me, my eyes would have slid shut as well.) Bikram yelled at LampPost and said that he would have to have a sit-down with Craig and himself to talk about things.

Bikram giveth, Bikram taketh.

THURSDAY 9 JUNE

# of days in yoga boot camp: 60
# of days until graduation: 2
# of hours til Prince arrives: 18

Our last day is tomorrow. Time is quite warpy. On one hand, I feel I've been here for a year. On the other hand, it feels like a week. Or a decade.

Bikram again used me as an example during lecture time. He joked that he now has my cold and that he cannot believe I worked so hard feeling so bad. Wow. King of Yogi apologizing. To moi. Little pear-shaped me. This is quite epic -- for both of us.

I sort of miss my anonymity. It is now impossible to nap or clean your toes when you know he might be calling out for you.

My cold is starting to clear. Morning class was really a struggle, I had to keep encouraging myself to stay in the damn room. Tonight's evening class with Craig was fun; our last class with him, in fact. Seems surreal that in 48 hours we will blow into the wind like fluffy dandelion seedlings.

Prince moved his flight so he'll be in early Friday—hooray! And!—Bikram has announced we will have no 7:30 A.M. Saturday class—he wants us to rest.

FRIDAY 10 JUNE

# of days in yoga boot camp: 61
# of days until graduation: 1
# of hours til Prince arrives: -2

Rajashree taught our morning class. The day was mostly a blur.

Our group has ended. Yesterday was really our last official day as a group. Lots of family coming in and lots of family taking the last class. Neighborhoods look funny with extra fence posts. Emily's Eddie arrives and takes class; I'm thrilled to meet him. Yet so sad that, like Mili, Emily will just vanish from my life and when I go to a Monday morning class, she just won't be there.

In the middle of Pranayama Breathing, Bikram's face appears over my mouth. How does he do that? Perhaps he is part Cobra.

He announces to the class: "I just looked in Miss Pink's mouth. Know what I see? Nails and rusty bolts. She very strong, Miss Pink. Know what I think? I think when she's dead, she will come back and chew on my toes at night, that's how strong Miss Pink is."

In Triangle, I pushed through the wicked hip pain and sat alllll the way down—and I felt almost as though I were floating. More tears streaming down my face. I look up at him and he's elsewhere, he's busy making fun of the family members.

Maybe he's set me free now—I no longer need his watchful eyes.

SATURDAY 11 JUNE

# of days in yoga boot camp: 62
# of days until graduation: 0

Mili came by around 10:30. Yay. I was worried, I didn't see her last night and couldn't find her apartment number; we'd promised all week we'd have pedicures in the morning.

I didn't really have anything cute to wear to graduation. I wanted to go shopping quickly. Mili convinced me to have a wash-and-style hair job instead of shopping. It seemed like an old-lady thing to do; have your hair styled before a party.

She put it into perspective.

"People always remember hair. You don't look at reunion pictures and say 'well, her top was boring' do you? No, you say 'Wow, did her hair turn out great.'"

Barely time to get my boring top on over my foofy hair—off to graduation.

Interesting to see the yoga studio room transformed into a nicer place, complete with a stage and a banner and chairs. No LampPost. Hard to fathom he won't graduate with us, it feels like a pinky finger has been cut off. Just to be sure, I scanned the program—his name was gone.

Comedy coach Sue came to graduation as well—such a nice treat. She sees Redhead Amy and her jaw drops and she says, "You know Amy?"

And before I can clarify, Sue says, "Is she here to perform?"

No, no, she's a yogi.

Sue seems incredulous that Amy would be a yogi and there's a weird disconnect.

"You don't know who she is, do you?"

Well, she drives a blue car and has green Ugg boots and wicked red hair and a very difficult family, plumbers I think.

"You don't recognize her from that show?"

No, I don't. I cannot fathom what Sue is getting at.

Amy comes up and we cannot believe that six-degrees-of-separation thing. That someone I took comedy class with a decade ago knows Amy.

I say to Prince that Sue recognized Amy. Prince laughs and says, "Well, she does look a lot like her father and her brother."

Doink.

I feel like an utter fool. Awfully famous family, and here I am, thinking they are Amish. Ohmygod, I offered to help her with comedy. Oh, god, she's in that one TV show, she's done a dozen movies, damnit, oh Ganesh, help me, I cannot face her ever again.

Most of the graduation ceremony was a blur. Leo the Bouncer was named our valedictorian, which made perfect sense. I kept thinking I couldn't believe I never put two and two together with Amy and I cannot believe LampPost is not graduating.

When I went up on stage to get my diploma, I heard some "Miss Pink" action from the crowd and then Bikram pointed at my shirt and said "Look, it is Miss Pink" and that warmed the cockles. Then my classmates cheered a little harder (I like to think) and it was glorious to feel like quite the celebrity for just those few moments.

I thought maybe it was a ruse or a game, maybe Bikram picks on one, ahem, well-proportioned gal each training. Either way, I wanted to thank him for showing me what humility is.

I also, although a little embarrassed at my slowness, admit to Bikram that on the last class on the last day of training, that in Triangle I did sit alllll the way down.

"I know, I saw you Miss Pink, you did good."

I told him that it finally felt like I was floating in the posture. Feeling like a fool, I blurt out "Bikram Yoga is so much easier than Miss Pink yoga."

Bikram grins ear to ear and burbles out "Can you believe it?"

He grabs my wrist, giving it a little tug, and pulls me closer to him.

"This is the best job in the world, Miss Pink. Don't ever forget that."

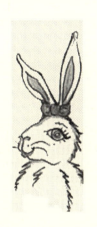

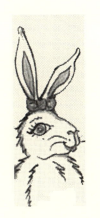

SPECIAL THANKS FOR REALLY SPECIAL PEOPLE

Candy & Charles: For nurturing the writer me for so very long.

Carol: If it weren't for you, I'd still be sitting in the lobby, rocking,
Clutching my manuscript.

Lockerroom Corner Girls: For making TT fun and goofy.

Danbury Dolphins: Teaching me to keep my head up whilst in deep, dark water. And – for beating the yoga drum.

DD: If it weren't for you, I'd still be rocking in the corner at Toe Stand.

Emily: Everything, everything, including the fine hare cut.

Erica: For that fabulous frozen water – and the faith therein.

Fran: Pulling that thin pink thread in my black years.

Frankie: The fabulous wonderful life-altering book title.

Friday 6:30 Gang: You all believing in me restored my lost faith.

Hilarie: So easily sharing your compassion and your teaching wisdom.

Karina: Goosing me to write that other book.

Katrina: Goosing me to finish this book.

Kellis: Goosing me (via Island Woods) to finish this book; not just this decade, but this year.

Kirsten: Anchoring my choppy waters, holding my hand those last two weeks.

Laura: Planting the teaching seed.

Mili: Your deep thoughts and cheery smile.

Monkey Butt: For making yoga boot camp just plain festive.

Rich Jaroslovsky: Setting me free, giving me a shove, telling me to "go find an audience."

Saiko: The upcoming Japanese Cobra Rabbit translation.

Seattle Cascades: So warmly embracing me as I relearned life (and synchro) skills.

Stewart: Really fine brownies ... and cornbread ... reminding me to nourish my soul.

Sue Peahl: Helping me find the fire -- and coaxing me to embrace the heat.

Tom: All the monkeys are so happy you coaxed them out of the attic in the first place.

Whoever I forgot: For your warm humor at my absentmindedness.

ABOUT THE AUTHOR

It is a little hard to imagine that you'd actually want to know more about me by now, assuming you've read through the book and didn't just skip to the end.

I live in the state of Washington with Prince and our two furry children, standard poodles Rebecca and Charley. I've hung my mat at Bikram Yoga Bellevue; I think it is the prettiest studio around. I practice and teach there when I'm not out on a book tour.

Prior to moving to the west coast, I spent a decade in New York City. Well, to be entirely truthful, I couldn't afford city rents, so I was always a Brooklyn gal. After Brooklyn, I spent many years in an old haunted farmhouse in Connecticut. Hauntings are not as fun as they sound -- do you have any idea how hard it is to keep a good electrician in your employ with spooks pulling their usual tricks?

Prior to the yoga teaching gig, I've worked in all sorts of fun jobs. For a while, I was the travel planner for the Dancing Raisins. Yes, I had mondo shoulder pads back then. I stumbled into Wall Street and worked with research analysts and traders. That stint led to financial journalism which led to radio which led to television which led to me wearing a lot of black and then bad things happened and then I wore pink sort of under duress and then I drove west and met Prince at a goofy singles party.

If you really crave more about my zany life, fear not. I've still got three more novels shoved in the back of one of these drawers. Visit me online for udpates and excerpts.

www.misspink.org

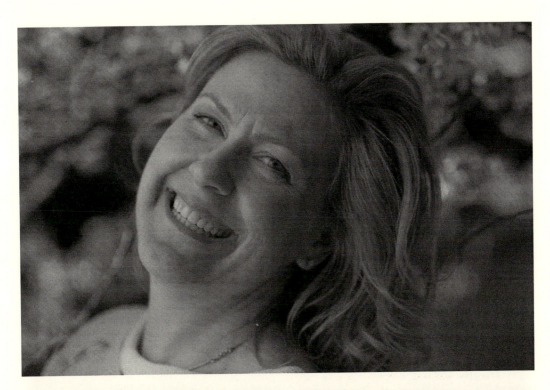

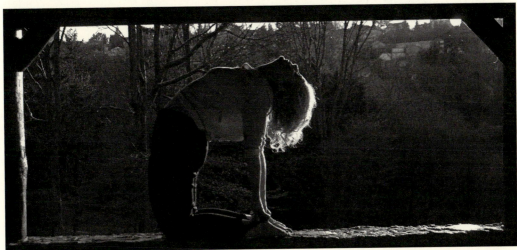

ABOUT THE ILLUSTRATOR

Teresa just made this book come to life. Initially, I had planned on typing up my notes from the yoga boot camp, going to Kinko's and mailing out the thing to my fellow boot camp survivors.

Several non-yoga friends said they liked the book, except for all the parts about the postures. Hmm.

Teresa went to teacher training with me -- she's the gal that had an artery in the front of her heart spontaneously tear. That's pretty much all I knew about her. As fate would have it, in the giant room of 200 people, I sat next to Teresa once. She was sketching faces for our yoga boot camp yearbook. I've always been in awe of people who can sing and people who can draw. Not only could she draw, but she was fast and the caricatures were spot-on.

I really wanted a visual aspect to this book, so I tentatively emailed Teresa. I'll admit, after nine weeks of that "the whole class will wait for Miss Pink" thing, I wasn't sure what kind of reception I'd get from Teresa.

I've been blown away and so wickedly blessed to have had Teresa scritch through my brain and bring everything to life, especially those precious monkeys.

When she wasn't busy trying to figure out how Shopping Monkey would dress, Teresa owns and manages a yoga studio in downtown Grapevine, Texas. She's married to a wonderfully loving husband and has 4 (four!) children ages 8 to 22. She's been illustrating for 15 years.

If you'd like more information on Teresa, visit her website at:
www.heartcenteredyogatx.com

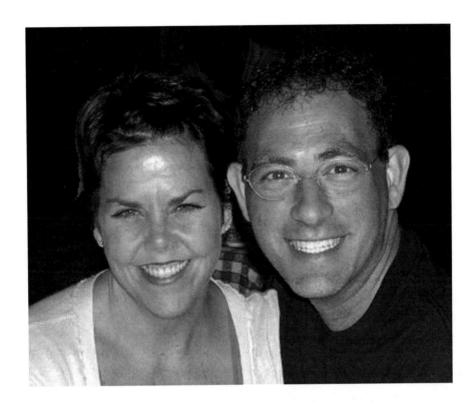

ABOUT THE COVER ARTIST

Marathon runners will tell you it is common to "hit the wall" around the 20th mile. There you are, plodding away, and then, wham!: no energy and you can no longer think straight.

My creative wall was the cover. The cover! The darn cover! I kept trying to distract myself by pawning the cover off on Teresa. But Teresa was busy dressing monkeys and putting finishing touches on the posture illustrations, and didn't fall for my tricks. I'll admit, I was a little flipped out. Books being judged by their covers and all.

Runners often rely on energy gel for the final miles. And that's what Jessica was for us – a zippy booster shot.

We knew for sure that Teresa's cobra and rabbit needed that je ne sais quoi. And Jessica was bright eyed and bushy tailed enough to see what we were too bleary to envision.

Jessica has been creating all sorts of fabulous art for 11 years. She does murals and faux floor coverings and real furniture. She currently lives in the Baltimore area and has a BFA in Children's Book Illustration.

For more information, feel free to stop by her website at:
www.jacartdesigns.com/pages

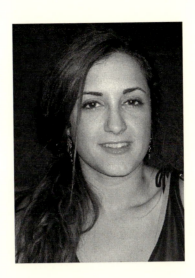

Made in the USA